Review of
DENTAL HYGIENE

Questions and Answers

PAULINE F. STEELE, B.S., R.D.H.,
B.S. (Educ.), M.A.

Director of Dental Hygiene and Associate Professor
University of Cincinnati

14 Contributors

35 Illustrations

Lea & Febiger

Philadelphia

To Ilse

PREFACE

The purpose of this book is to provide for the hygienist an authoritative source of review. Today, there is a continuing accumulation of knowledge in every discipline, as well as an increasing need for the standardization of examinations that test proficiency. It is hoped, therefore, that this work will prove to be a useful review of all the subjects studied by dental hygienists.

Although there are a variety of patterns that can be utilized to review previously learned material, an effective approach is the proposal of hypothetical questions. This process encourages the student to consider the original principle involved, stimulates recall of facts, and exemplifies their applicability to a particular situation. This book is not intended merely to provide facts, but also to encourage the student to arrive at answers through sound reasoning. Only with considerable difficulty can it be established where rote memorization ends and methodical reasoning begins. However, before the problem solving technique is possible, both of these abilities must exist.

The contributors to this work are specialists in the field and are directly associated with dental hygiene education. In every chapter major emphasis is placed on fundamental concepts and pertinent facts, in order to facilitate a philosophically reflective study of the subject. This objective is in direct contrast to the belief that a review book should be a reiteration of every statement made during a course. To paraphrase a famous philosopher: Knowledge without data is worthless, while data without understanding is meaningless.

Special acknowledgment is accorded each contributor for the excellent material submitted. Only through such concerted interest and splendid cooperation has the realization of this effort been possible. It is hoped that this book will be a beneficial educational contribution for the dental hygienist.

PAULINE F. STEELE

Cincinnati, Ohio

CONTRIBUTORS

Camillo A. Alberico, D.D.S., M.S.
Associate Professor, School of Dentistry,
West Virginia University, Morgantown, West Virginia

Henry W. Aplington, Jr., B.A., M.A., Ph.D.
Professor of Anatomy, College of Medicine,
Ohio State University, Columbus, Ohio

Katharine K. Aplington, B.A., M.A.
Instructor in Anatomy, School of Medicine,
Ohio State University, Columbus, Ohio

Carroll G. Bennett, B.S., D.D.S., M.S. (Physiology)
Professor and Chairman, Department of Pedodontics,
School of Dentistry, West Virginia University,
Morgantown, West Virginia

Harold H. Boyers, D.D.S.
Associate Professor, School of Dentistry,
West Virginia University, Morgantown, West Virginia

C. Keith Claycomb, B.S., M.S., Ph.D.
Professor and Chairman, Department of Biochemistry,
University of Oregon, School of Dentistry, Portland, Oregon

Babette Graf, B.S., M.S.
Assistant Professor of Nutrition, and Institutional Administration,
West Virginia University, Morgantown, West Virginia

Elmer E. Kelln, B.S., D.D.S., M.S.D. (Pathology), F.A.C.D.
Associate Professor, School of Dentistry, Loma Linda University;
Coordinator of Hospital Dental Services, Orange County General
Hospital, Los Angeles, California

JAMES OVERBERGER, B.S., D.D.S., M.S.
Associate Professor of Prosthodontics, School of Dentistry,
University of North Carolina, Chapel Hill, North Carolina

DOROTHY PERMAR, B.S., M.S.
Associate Professor, School of Dentistry,
Ohio State University, Columbus, Ohio

DORIS O. POWLEN, A.B., M.S.
Associate in Microbiology, School of Dental Medicine,
University of Pennsylvania, Philadelphia, Pennsylvania

NANCY J. REYNOLDS, D.D.S.
Associate Professor, School of Dentistry,
Ohio State University, Columbus, Ohio

EDITH R. SANDERS, B.S., R.D.H., M.P.H.
Instructor, School of Dentistry,
University of Kentucky, Lexington, Kentucky

PAULINE F. STEELE, B.S., B.Sc., R.D.H., M.A.
Associate Professor and Director of Dental Hygiene,
University of Cincinnati, Cincinnati, Ohio

RUTH R. SWORDS, B.A., B.S., D.D.S.
Professor and Director of Dental Hygiene,
Caruth School of Dental Hygiene, Baylor University, Dallas, Texas

CONTENTS

CHAPTER 1

HISTOLOGY AND EMBRYOLOGY

Dorothy Permar

1. In the early embryo, there are three primary embryonic layers (germ layers). Some of the structures derived from the outer layer, the *ectoderm*, include the

   a. brain, nails, tooth enamel, epithelium of the gingival mucosa, and epithelium of the nasal chamber
   b. brain, hair, papillae of the body of the tongue, and epithelium and connective tissue of the gingival mucosa
   c. nails, tooth enamel, epithelium of the skin, and the entire mucous membrane of the anterior part of the mouth
   d. nails, hair, epithelium of the pharynx, epithelium of the esophagus, and epithelium of the skin

2. Some of the structures derived from the middle primary embryonic layer, the *mesoderm*, include the

   a. muscles, nervous system, blood system, and epithelium lining the digestive tract
   b. muscles, blood, skeleton, and brain
   c. heart muscle, nervous system, dentin, and tooth pulp
   d. muscles, skeleton, dentin, and connective tissue of the oral mucosa

3. Some of the structures derived from the inner primary embryonic layer, the *endoderm*, include the

   a. kidneys, blood, nerves, and epithelial lining of the intestines
   b. dentin, tooth pulp, connective tissue of the oral mucosa, and epithelial lining of the lungs
   c. epithelial lining of the lungs, epithelial lining of the stomach, and epithelial lining of the pharynx
   d. tooth pulp, tooth enamel, epithelial lining of the trachea, and epithelial lining of the pharynx

4. The earliest sign of development of the human face occurs during the
   third week in utero with the formation of the

   a. stomodeum
   b. nasal openings
   c. maxillary processes of the second branchial arch
   d. fourth branchial arch

5. The buccopharyngeal membrane is composed of

   a. mesoderm and endoderm
   b. ectoderm and mesoderm
   c. ectoderm, mesoderm, and endoderm
   d. endoderm and ectoderm

6. In the embryonic development of the oral and nasal cavities, the
   structures that develop from the depression known as the stomodeum
   include the

   a. mouth cavity, body and base of the tongue, and nasal chamber
   b. mouth cavity, nasal chamber, and maxillary sinuses
   c. nasal cavity, pharynx, and body of the tongue
   d. nasal cavity, pharynx, and hard palate

7. In the embryonic development of the face and oral cavity, the first
   branchial arch gives rise to the

   a. base of the tongue, mandible, lateral parts of the hard palate,
      and the soft palate
   b. body of the tongue, only the anterior 1/3 of the hard palate,
      and mandible
   c. body of the tongue, mandible, all but the anterior part of the
      palate, and nasal septum
   d. sides of the hard palate, soft palate, body of the tongue, and
      mandible

8. The frontal process of the early embryo gives rise, ultimately, to the

   a. center of the nose, sides of the upper lip, maxillary processes,
      and nasal septum
   b. center of the nose, sides of the nose, nasal septum, premaxilla,
      and center of the upper lip
   c. median nasal process, lateral nasal processes, maxillary proc-
      esses, and globular process
   d. median nasal process, brain, nasal septum, and most of the hard
      palate

9. In the embryonic development of the upper lip, a cleft will result if there is a failure of proper fusion between the

    a. maxillary processes and premaxilla
    b. right and left maxillary processes
    c. globular process and a maxillary process
    d. lateral nasal process and maxillary process

10. In the embryonic development of the oral cavity, area C in Figure 1 is a derivative of the

    a. first branchial arch
    b. frontal process
    c. median nasal process
    d. second branchial arch

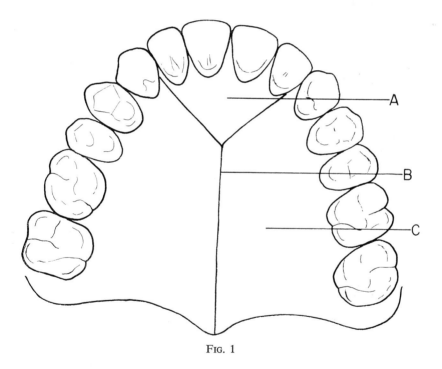

FIG. 1

11. In the embryonic development of the oral cavity, line B in Figure 1 is ordinarily completely fused by the end of the

    a. fifth month in utero
    b. third month in utero
    c. fourth week in utero
    d. sixth week in utero

12. In the embryonic development of the oral cavity, the origin of area A in Figure 1 is the

   a. first branchial arch
   b. lateral nasal processes
   c. frontal process
   d. maxillary processes

13. In the development of the oral cavity, the fusions of the embryonic processes which form the roof of the mouth are usually completed by the

   a. end of the fifth month in utero
   b. end of the fifth week in utero
   c. end of the second month in utero
   d. end of the third month in utero

14. In the embryonic development of the face, a reduction in the size of the mouth results from fusion between the

   a. mandibular arch and maxillary processes
   b. right and left maxillary processes
   c. premaxillary and maxillary processes
   d. first and second branchial arches

15. The composition of epithelial tissues is characterized by

   a. much intercellular substance and few cells
   b. no intercellular substance
   c. little intercellular substance in proportion to the number of cells
   d. intercellular substance in the surface layer only

16. Simple squamous epithelial cells are found

   a. lining blood vessels and lymphatic ducts
   b. lining the nasal cavity
   c. on the lower surface of the tongue
   d. lining the trachea

17. Ciliated columnar epithelium *or* ciliated pseudostratified epithelium is found in the

   a. trachea, nasal cavity, esophagus, urinary bladder, and lungs
   b. trachea, nasal cavity, maxillary sinuses, bronchi, and fallopian tubes
   c. trachea, nasal cavity, maxillary sinuses, and stomach
   d. trachea, nasal cavity, lining of larger arteries, and fallopian tubes

18. The fibers of connective tissue proper are classified as

   a. collagenous, muscular, elastic, and reticular
   b. reticular, elastic, and collagenous
   c. collagenous, mesenchymal, elastic, and fibrous
   d. elastic, longitudinal, reticular, and collagenous

19. The skin on the palm of the hand is composed of an epidermis and a corium. The epidermis consists of

   a. stratum corneum, stratum lucidum, stratum granulosum, stratum germinativum, and striated muscle
   b. stratum corneum, stratum lucidum, stratum germinativum, and smooth muscle layer
   c. stratum corneum, stratum lucidum, stratum granulosum containing hair follicles, and stratum germinativum
   d. stratum corneum, stratum lucidum, stratum granulosum, and stratum germinativum

20. A mucous membrane is found lining

   a. the stomach, the abdominal wall, and the intestines
   b. the mouth, the thorax, the esophagus, and the intestines
   c. any body cavity that opens to the outside of the body
   d. the mouth, the stomach, the liver, and the lungs

21. A mucous membrane is composed of

   a. epithelium, either stratified squamous, simple squamous, or columnar
   b. epithelium and connective tissue
   c. epithelium, underlying connective tissue, and minute muscle fibers
   d. epithelium, nerves, lymphatic vessels, blood vessels, and striated muscle fibers

22. Assume that you have a description of an organ which includes the following terms: nephron, Bowman's capsule, loop of Henle, glomeruli, convoluted tubule, cortex, medulla. You know from these terms that the described organ is the

   a. spleen
   b. liver
   c. pancreas
   d. kidney

23. The cells of the blood are of different types. The types include

    a. erythrocytes, polymorphonuclear erythrocytes, polymorphonuclear basophils, polymorphonuclear monocytes, and polymorphonuclear neutrophils
    b. erythrocytes, eosinophils, basophils, neurocytes, polymorphonuclear neutrophils, and lymphocytes
    c. polymorphonuclear neutrophils, basophils, eosinophils, monocytes, and erythrocytes
    d. eosinophils, polymorphonuclear erythrocytes, basophils, polymorphonuclear neutrophils, monocytes, and lymphocytes

24. In the adult body, the different types of blood cells are normally formed in the following locations:

    a. erythrocytes and eosinophils in red bone marrow, and lymphocytes and basophils in lymph nodules
    b. red blood cells and lymphocytes in the alveolar process, and eosinophils and basophils in the spleen
    c. erythrocytes and granulocytes in red bone marrow, and lymphocytes in lymph nodules
    d. monocytes and neutrophils in the lymph nodules, and granulocytes and lymphocytes in red bone marrow

25. Hemopoietic tissue may be described as

    a. a specialized tissue derived from endoderm which produces different kinds of white blood cells
    b. yellow bone marrow which produces new blood cells and removes old blood cells from the blood stream
    c. connective tissue which is highly specialized to produce new blood cells and remove worn-out blood cells from the blood stream
    d. a specialized endothelial tissue which produces erythrocytes

26. The type of muscle referred to as smooth muscle is found in different places in the body. These places include the

    a. wall of the intestine, wall of the stomach, wall of the ureter, wall of the urinary bladder, walls of blood vessels
    b. walls of blood vessels, wall of the intestine, marginal gingiva, and wall of the ureter
    c. wall of the urinary bladder, adrenal cortex, walls of the large and small intestines, and wall of the stomach
    d. walls of blood vessels, half of the heart muscle, cerebellum, and walls of the intestines and stomach

27. Cartilage tissue occurs in three forms which are known as

    a. fibrous, osseous, and hyaline
    b. elastic, nonelastic, and osseous
    c. hyaline, osseous, and elastic
    d. fibrous, hyaline, and elastic

28. Dendrites and axons are collectively called

    a. nerve cells
    b. synapses
    c. perikaryons
    d. nerve fibers

29. Neurons which convey impulses to muscles or glands, stimulating them to action, are called

    a. association neurons
    b. motor neurons
    c. sensory neurons
    d. reflex neurons

30. In the nasal cavity, most of the epithelial lining is composed of

    a. stratified squamous epithelium that is not keratinized
    b. pseudostratified ciliated columnar epithelium and goblet cells
    c. stratified squamous epithelium that is keratinized
    d. stratified ciliated columnar epithelium and cuboidal cells

31. The types of epithelium found in the lining of the oral cavity include

    a. simple squamous and stratified squamous
    b. keratinized and nonkeratinized stratified squamous
    c. stratified cuboidal and stratified squamous
    d. keratinized stratified squamous and nonkeratinized simple squamous

32. In the oral cavity, one way in which lining mucosa differs from masticatory mucosa is that

    a. lining mucosa has glands beneath it and masticatory mucosa has fat tissue beneath it
    b. lining mucosa lines the inside of the mouth and masticatory mucosa masticates the food
    c. lining mucosa is nonkeratinized and masticatory mucosa usually has a keratin layer
    d. lining mucosa contains more muscle fibers than masticatory mucosa

33. In contrast to the *masticatory mucosa*, the areas of oral mucosa classified as *lining mucosa* include the

    a. lips, cheeks, alveolar mucosa, gingival mucosa, floor of the mouth, underside of the tongue, and soft palate
    b. cheeks, alveolar mucosa, dorsum of the tongue, floor of the mouth, and soft palate
    c. inside of the lips, cheeks, palatine raphe, floor of the mouth, and undersurface of the tongue
    d. undersurface of the tongue, lips, cheeks, soft palate, and floor of the mouth

34. The type of epithelium lining the inside of the cheeks is

    a. stratified, nonkeratinized columnar
    b. keratinized, stratified squamous
    c. nonkeratinized, stratified pseudosquamous
    d. nonkeratinized, stratified squamous

35. One of the ways in which the gingival mucosa and the mucosa of the hard palate differ is that

    a. the gingival mucosa is keratinized and the palatal mucosa is not keratinized
    b. the gingival mucosa has underlying it glands of a different type from those of the palatal mucosa
    c. the gingival mucosa has no glands or fat underlying it and the palatal mucosa has glands and fat underlying most of it
    d. the gingival mucosa has epithelial cells of a type considerably different from those of the palatal mucosa

36. The connective tissue part of the oral mucosa is composed chiefly of

    a. fibrous connective tissue, minute muscle fibers, and fat cells
    b. minute muscle fibers in which are nerves and blood vessels
    c. fibrous connective tissue in which are blood vessels and nerves
    d. mesoderm, smooth muscle fibers, nerves, and blood vessels

37. The tongue has on it many papillae of different kinds. The kinds of papillae may include

    a. circumvallate, circumfoliate, fungiform, and fusiform
    b. circumvallate, fungiform, filiform, and foliate
    c. fungiform, fusiform, and circumvallate
    d. circumvallate, filiform, and fatty

38. Fordyce's spots are a result of

    a. overdevelopment of circumvallate papillae of the tongue
    b. entrapping of sebaceous glands in the embryonic fusion of the maxillary processes and the mandibular arch
    c. inflammation of fungiform papillae of the tongue
    d. drops of enamel having been formed on the root of a tooth, particularly the mandibular molars

39. The secretory elements of the major salivary glands (parotid, submandibular, sublingual) are composed of

    a. specialized cells derived from the mesenchyme of the oral cavity
    b. specialized cells derived from endoderm
    c. ingrowths from remnants of the buccopharyngeal membrane
    d. specialized cells derived from ectoderm

40. The parotid glands empty into the oral cavity through the parotid ducts. The openings of these ducts are located

    a. opposite the mandibular first molars
    b. opposite the maxillary first premolars
    c. opposite the maxillary second molars
    d. under the tongue

41. After the tooth crown has emerged into the oral cavity, the part of the reduced enamel epithelium which remains surrounding the cervical part of the crown is henceforth referred to as the

    a. gingival epithelium
    b. marginal gingiva
    c. enamel cuticle
    d. epithelium of the gingival sulcus and the epithelial attachment

42. One change in the epithelial attachment that ordinarily occurs as the individual ages is

    a. the epithelial attachment moves apically on the tooth
    b. the epithelial attachment becomes keratinized
    c. the epithelial attachment becomes cemented to the crown
    d. the epithelial attachment is converted into connective tissue

43. In a young person of about 10 years of age, the location of the apical end of the epithelial attachment of the maxillary central incisor teeth probably would be

    a. about 1 mm from the apex of the root
    b. approximately at the cementoenamel junction
    c. on the enamel, about 1 mm incisal to the cementoenamel junction
    d. near the cervical line on the mesial surface, and about 3 mm apical to this on the distal surface

44. The presence of large amounts of calculus in the gingival sulcus may be expected to

   a. damage the epithelium of the gingival sulcus, cause resorption of the root apex, and cause formation of excessive cementum at the apex
   b. damage the gingival group of periodontal ligament fibers, produce additional dentin formation beneath the periodontal ligament, and produce inflammation of the gingival tissue
   c. produce inflammation of the gingival tissue, produce caries beneath the calculus, and result in resorption of the bone of the alveolar crest
   d. damage the epithelium of the gingival sulcus, produce inflammation and swelling of the adjacent gingiva, damage the fibers of the periodontal ligament in the inflamed area, and result in resorption of the bone of the alveolar crest

45. In a 10-year-old child, it is to be expected that the size of the clinical root of the right maxillary central incisor tooth will be

   a. larger than the anatomic root
   b. smaller than the anatomic root
   c. the same size as the anatomic root
   d. smaller than the clinical crown

46. The calcified tissues of a tooth listed in the order of decreasing hardness are

   a. enamel, cementum, dentin, interglobular dentin
   b. enamel, interglobular dentin, dentin, cementum
   c. dentin, enamel, cementum
   d. enamel, dentin, cementum

47. In human enamel, each enamel rod is encased in

   a. a hypercalcified coating
   b. a gelatinous protective covering
   c. a rod sheath
   d. nothing

48. The average diameter of an enamel rod in a human tooth is approximately

   a. 25 microns
   b. 4 microns
   c. 0.25 millimeter
   d. 1 micron

49. In a fissure on the occlusal surface of a tooth, the enamel rods that line the fissure are so oriented that their position is approximately

    a. parallel to the dentinoenamel junction
    b. perpendicular to the walls of the fissure
    c. perpendicular to the dentinoenamel junction
    d. circular, around the curvature of the fissure, and parallel to its exposed surface

50. Enamel tufts are composed of

    a. peripheral ends of dentinal fibers
    b. brush-like structures in the enamel which are hypercalcified
    c. protrusions of dentinal tubules into the enamel
    d. inner ends of enamel rods (ends nearest the dentin) which are poorly calcified

51. An enamel spindle is composed of

    a. cytoplasm of a specialized pulp cell
    b. a poorly calcified enamel rod
    c. poorly calcified interrod substance
    d. an end of a dentinal tubule

52. The mineral substance in mature enamel exists in the form of

    a. a nonmolecular mass
    b. submicroscopic crystals
    c. an inorganic membrane
    d. a metallic sheet

53. The mineral contents of enamel and of dentin are, respectively, approximately

    a. 96% and 70%
    b. 80% and 70%
    c. 100% and 70%
    d. 90% and 50%

54. To say that the enamel of a tooth shows *attrition* means that

    a. it has conspicuous horizontal formation lines on the facial surface
    b. it is worn off as a result of meeting opposing teeth with sufficient force for a sufficiently long period of time
    c. it has visible vertical cracks on the facial surface
    d. it has become slightly discolored with age

55. The condition of exposed cervical cementum often found in older persons frequently is accompanied by

      a. a marked cervical attrition of the enamel
      b. an apical extension of Tomes' granular layer
      c. abrasion of the cementum on the facial surfaces of the teeth
      d. an additional covering of the epithelial attachment

56. Excluding from consideration the dentinal fibers that occupy the dentinal tubules, dentin is composed of

      a. fibrils, interrod substance, cementing substance, and crystallized minerals
      b. fibrils, cementing substance, and mineral substance in crystalline form
      c. organic cementing substance, minerals, and interrod substance
      d. dentinal processes, fibrils, cementing substance, and crystallized minerals

57. Sometimes certain areas of dentin are said to be *sclerotic.* This means that

      a. the dentin has become slightly decalcified
      b. this area of dentin contains the bacteria which produce caries
      c. the dentin in this area has become bone-like
      d. the dentinal tubules have become filled with mineral substances

58. Some dentin is referred to, histologically, as *secondary dentin,* which is *best* described as

      a. dentin produced in later life, usually with tubules bent more or less sharply at the line of separation between it and earlier dentin, and sometimes with irregularly arranged tubules
      b. dentin produced secondarily which is less calcified and softer than the original dentin
      c. dentin produced as a result of caries, containing more dentinal fibers and more branched tubules than ordinary dentin, and being more highly calcified than ordinary dentin
      d. dentin in which the dentinal tubules have become obliterated by deposition of mineral substances

59. The Tomes' fibers which occupy the dentinal tubules are part of

      a. the Korff's fibers of the pulp
      b. the odontoblasts of the pulp
      c. the fibrillar dentin matrix
      d. the interrod substance of the dentin

60. *Interglobular dentin* is best described as

    a. empty spaces in dentin between globules

    b. dentin with irregular tubules between globules of normal dentin

    c. small areas in the dentin which are uncalcified or less calcified than the remainder of the dentin of that tooth, usually located in a band in the crown some distance inside the dentinoenamel junction, and sometimes in the root some distance inside the dentinocemental junction

    d. dentin that is produced in globules during the development of the tooth

61. Tooth pulp contains several kinds of cells. Among the cells commonly found in healthy young tooth pulp are

    a. fibroblasts, osteoblasts, odontoblasts, histiocytes, and undifferentiated mesenchymal cells

    b. odontoblasts, denticles, leukocytes, fibroblasts, and ameloblasts

    c. histiocytes, fibroblasts, undifferentiated mesenchymal cells, odontoblasts, and erythrocytes

    d. fibroblasts, goblet cells, erythrocytes, undifferentiated mesenchymal cells, and odontoblasts

62. Functions of the pulp include

    a. sensory function for both dentin and cementum, formation of dentin, calcification of cementum, and defense reactions

    b. formation of dentin and cementum, defense against bacterial invasion, and supplying blood to cementum

    c. resorption of cementum, alteration of dentin to sclerotic dentin, nutritive function, and sensory function for both pulp and dentin

    d. formation of dentin, sensory function for both pulp and dentin, nutritive function, and defense reactions against mechanical or chemical stimuli or bacterial invasion

63. Dentinal fibers (Tomes' fibers) are composed of

    a. fibrous bundles enclosed in the dentinal tubules

    b. fibrils from the dentin matrix extending through the dentinal tubules

    c. cytoplasmic extensions of pulp cells extending through the dentin toward the dentinoenamel or dentinocemental junction

    d. muscular fibers extending from pulp cells to the dentinoenamel junction

64. Among the structures which ordinarily may be found in tooth pulp are

   a. blood vessels, lymph vessels, nerves, Korff's fibers, and diffuse calcifications
   b. blood vessels, nerves, Korff's fibers, Sharpey's fibers, and denticles
   c. nerves, dentinal spindles, blood vessels, and lymph vessels
   d. Korff's fibers, denticles, nerves, lacunae, and blood vessels

65. The pulp of a newly formed tooth and the pulp of a tooth of an elderly person do not present the same macroscopic or microscopic picture. They differ in that the older pulp

   a. often contains more and larger denticles; is slightly larger due to loss of dentin, with a consequent increase in size of the pulp chamber; contains fewer blood vessels
   b. has an increased blood supply; has fewer cells and more fibrous intercellular substance; has diffuse calcifications
   c. is smaller due to a decrease in the size of the pulp chamber; contains fewer cells; contains more fibrous intercellular substance; contains fewer blood vessels
   d. often has large denticles; has fewer cells; often contains specialized osteoblasts; contains more fibrous substance

66. Tomes' granular layer is best described as

   a. a band of granules of dentin in the tooth root beneath the cementum
   b. a layer of sensitive granular cementum near the root apex
   c. a band of minute uncalcified or poorly calcified areas in the root dentin very close to the cementum
   d. a layer of areas of sensitive uncalcified dentin extending around the outer portion of the dentin beneath the cementum of the root and the enamel of the crown of the tooth

67. The location and direction of the lines of Retzius may be correctly described as being

   a. in the enamel, approximately perpendicular to the dentinoenamel junction
   b. in the dentin, following the contour of the dentinoenamel junction
   c. in the alveolar bone, parallel to the surface adjoining the periodontal ligament
   d. in the enamel, extending outward from the dentinoenamel junction toward the occlusal, or incisal, part of the crown

68. Perikymata on teeth are said to be related to

    a. delayed eruption of the tooth
    b. lines of Retzius
    c. irregular lines in the dentin
    d. poor calcification of the dentin

69. The structures on teeth called *mamelons* are

    a. abnormalities due to faulty dentin formation
    b. lobes due to improper formation of the outer enamel epithelium
    c. lobes on the incisal edges of anterior teeth
    d. abnormalities of enamel due to malnutrition

70. The bands of Hunter-Schreger, as seen under a microscope by reflected light, are a result of

    a. branching of dentinal tubules
    b. differences in light reflection due to changes in direction of the enamel rods
    c. a nutritional deficiency during the period of tooth development
    d. hypercalcification of the interrod substances

71. From which primary embryonic layer or layers is an enamel spindle derived?

    a. ectoderm
    b. endoderm
    c. mesoderm
    d. ectoderm and mesoderm

72. Bone tissue consists of

    a. osteoblasts, fibrous and amorphous intercellular substance, and mineral material
    b. mineral substance, fibrous and amorphous intercellular substance, lamellae, osteoclasts, and Haversian systems
    c. Volkmann's canals, marrow space, canaliculi, cartilage cells, and blood vessels
    d. osteocytes, fibrous and amorphous intercellular substance, and mineral substance

73. *Osteocytes* are connected to one another by means of

    a. fibrils extending from the nuclei of each cell
    b. blood vessels which extend from lacuna to lacuna through canaliculi
    c. nothing at all; there is no connection
    d. connecting extensions of their cytoplasm which are located in canaliculi

74. *Osteoclasts* are associated with the process of
    a. the nutrition and maintenance of bone tissue
    b. the production of bone tissue in the mandible
    c. the resorption, or removal, of calcified bone tissue
    d. the apposition of bone tissue in Haversian systems

75. *Osteoblasts* may be correctly described as
    a. multinucleated connective tissue cells which are associated with bone resorption
    b. connective tissue cells which are associated with bone apposition
    c. connective tissue cells specialized to function in the decalcification of bone
    d. endothelial cells surrounding forming bone tissue

76. The process of growth of a bone includes
    a. bone apposition and bone resorption, but neither decalcification nor cell division of the osteocytes
    b. bone apposition, bone decalcification, bone resorption
    c. bone apposition, cell division of osteocytes, bone resorption
    d. bone apposition, division of osteocytes, and matrix mineralization

77. To speak of *endochondral formation of bone* means that
    a. cartilage becomes bone as it matures
    b. a cartilage structure which precedes the bone tissue becomes calcified and is resorbed, and is replaced by bone tissue
    c. a bone forms with a cartilage covering for protection, and the covering later resorbs
    d. bone tissue forms around a large blood vessel, with cartilage on the inner surface

78. To speak of *intramembranous formation of bone* means that
    a. bone matrix forms and calcifies in connective tissue without being preceded by cartilage formation
    b. bone forms with a muscular membrane surrounding it which produces and resorbs the tissue
    c. bone forms first as a thin membrane and is then converted into bone
    d. bone matrix has a membrane running through it in layers

79. The cells which are associated with bone apposition and bone resorption are, respectively,
    a. osteocytes and osteums
    b. osteoclasts and osteoblasts
    c. osteoids and osteocoels
    d. osteoblasts and osteoclasts

80. The term *endosteum* is applied to

    a. the fibrous, organic membrane between layers of bone
    b. the connective tissue covering all inside surfaces of a bone
    c. the connective tissue around the outside of a bone that produces new bone
    d. the lining of the lacunae of bone tissue

81. The pattern of arrangement of the bone tissue in a Haversian system is

    a. in concentric lamellae around central canals
    b. in no special arrangement, but is perforated by Haversian canals
    c. in diagonal layers between Haversian systems
    d. in layers of bone tissue which follow the outline of the marrow cavity

82. Haversian canals in bone tissue are lined with

    a. periosteum
    b. endothelial cells
    c. endosteum
    d. endochondral cells

83. Subperiosteal bone is found

    a. around the outer layer of every Haversian system
    b. lining the bone marrow cavity
    c. on the outside surface of a bone immediately beneath the periosteum
    d. beneath the periosteum of all cartilage

84. The alveolar process is composed of

    a. a very hard tissue in the alveolar bone proper (also called lamina dura, or true alveolar bone), a softer bone tissue in the cortical plate, and a much less calcified trabecular bone between the two
    b. solid Haversian system type bone between the lamina dura and the cortical plate
    c. an inner layer called alveolar bone proper (lamina dura, true alveolar bone), and an outer supporting structure composed of (a) the cortical plate and (b) in some areas of the mouth an intervening trabecular type bone
    d. a combination of bone, cartilage, and cementum

85. The bone marrow cavity of an adult human mandible ordinarily may be expected to contain

    a. fat cells, blood vessels, considerable amounts of red bone marrow, nerves, and trabeculae
    b. trabeculae, lymph vessels, fat cells, denticles, and nerves
    c. blood vessels, chondrocytes, some red bone marrow, some yellow bone marrow, and nerves
    d. blood vessels, nerves, very little if any red bone marrow, fat cells, and trabeculae

86. The periodontal ligament is attached to

    a. true alveolar bone (lamina dura) and dentin
    b. cementum and trabecular bone
    c. cementum and cervical enamel
    d. cementum and lamina dura

87. Structures that are often found in the periodontal ligament include

    a. fibers, blood vessels, denticles, nerves, osteoclasts, and cementoblasts
    b. osteoclasts, epithelial cells, cementicles, blood vessels, fibers, and lymph vessels
    c. nerves, lymph vessels, osteocytes, denticles, fibers, and cells
    d. cementicles, blood vessels, muscles, fibers, nerves, and osteoblasts

88. The width of the periodontal ligament has been found to be approximately in the range of

    a. 1 to 5 millimeters
    b. 2 to 3 millimeters
    c. 0.12 to 0.33 millimeters
    d. 1.6 to 1.8 millimeters

89. The functions performed by the periodontal ligament include

    a. support of the tooth in the alveolus, cementum apposition, bone apposition, cementum and bone resorption, and sensitivity to pressure on the tooth
    b. support of the tooth in the alveolus, cementum apposition, dentin apposition, bone apposition, and resorption of cementum and bone
    c. formation of the lamina dura (true alveolar bone), resorption of cementum, attachment to cortical plate, and prevention of excessive tooth tilting
    d. attachment of cervical gingiva to the tooth, resorption of the tooth root, apposition of dentin, and support of the tooth in the alveolus

90. The structures in the periodontal ligament ordinarily referred to as the *free gingival fibers* have ends of the fibers attached

    a. to the alveolar bone and to the cementum
    b. to the cementum and to the epithelium of the gingiva
    c. to the cementum and into the connective tissue of the gingiva near its cervical border
    d. to the enamel and to the free gingiva

91. The structures in the periodontal ligament ordinarily referred to as the *transseptal fibers* are attached by their ends to

    a. the cementum of adjacent teeth and the alveolar crest between these teeth
    b. the cementum of proximal surfaces of adjacent teeth cervical to the alveolar crest between the teeth
    c. the cementum on the mesial or distal root surfaces of a tooth and to the alveolar bone opposite
    d. the cortical plate and across the free gingiva

92. The earliest sign of human tooth development is found in the anterior mandibular region at the embryonic age of about

    a. 5 to 6 months
    b. 5 to 6 days
    c. 3 to 4 months
    d. 5 to 6 weeks

93. The dental lamina may be described as

    a. an ingrowth of oral endoderm which gives rise to the dentin and cementum of the developing tooth
    b. a layer of oral mesenchyme from which the tooth pulp is derived as the tooth develops
    c. a layer of hypertrophied tissue found along the gingival margin in certain types of disease
    d. a band of thickened oral epithelium extending along the occlusal borders of the embryonic jaws from which arises the epithelial part of the tooth germ

94. All of the tissues and organs of the body are derived from ectoderm, mesoderm, endoderm, or some combination of these.

    Tooth enamel is derived from

    a. mesoderm and ectoderm
    b. endoderm and mesoderm
    c. endoderm
    d. ectoderm

Dentin is derived from

    a. ectoderm
    b. endoderm
    c. mesoderm
    d. mesoderm and endoderm

Cementum is derived from

    a. endoderm
    b. endoderm and mesoderm
    c. mesoderm
    d. ectoderm

95. The *epithelium of the mucosa* lining the inside of the lips is derived from

    a. endoderm
    b. ectoderm
    c. endoderm and mesoderm
    d. ectoderm and mesoderm

96. In the development of a tooth, the structure called the dental sac is a derivative of

    a. the dental lamina
    b. mesoderm (or mesenchyme)
    c. ectoderm
    d. the mandibular or maxillary bone

97. The dental sac gives rise to the

    a. outer layer of tooth pulp
    b. structure that encloses the functioning tooth crown
    c. periodontal ligament
    d. enamel cuticle

98. In the development of a permanent tooth, the time that the root formation is completed is about

    a. the time the tooth emerges into the oral cavity
    b. two to three months after the tooth emerges
    c. a year after the tooth emerges
    d. one to four years after the tooth emerges

99. In a tooth germ at the stage of development which immediately precedes the beginning of hard tissue formation, the line of union between the ameloblasts and odontoblasts is approximately the configuration of the future

    a. outside surface of the tooth crown
    b. cementoenamel junction
    c. dentinoenamel junction
    d. inner wall of the pulp chamber

100. Hertwig's epithelial root sheath may be described as

    a. a network of cells in the periodontal ligament composed of epithelial cells which are the remains of the inner and outer enamel epithelium
    b. a sheath of cells which snugly fits the outer surface of the cementum and attaches it to the periodontal ligament
    c. a band of epithelial cells around the cervical portion of the roots of older teeth
    d. a layer of epithelial cells which sometimes forms about a tooth root in certain conditions of disease and causes the teeth to become loose

101. The enamel organs of all tooth germs develop from the dental lamina. The enamel organs of the tooth germs of *certain* permanent teeth develop from the dental lamina lingual to the tooth germs of certain deciduous teeth. Of the *permanent teeth* listed below, the enamel organs develop from the dental lamina lingual to a deciduous tooth in

    a. all incisors, canines, and first molars
    b. all incisors, canines, and premolars
    c. all permanent teeth
    d. the permanent molar teeth

102. Tooth eruption begins at the time

    a. the first dentin is produced
    b. the root is completed
    c. the root begins to form
    d. the hard tissues become calcified

103. The normal events which finally result in the shedding of a deciduous maxillary molar tooth are

    a. the deciduous tooth roots undergo a continuous, very slow resorption owing to the presence of the developing permanent molars

    b. the deciduous tooth roots are resorbed one at a time, beginning usually with the mesiobuccal root; the developing permanent tooth which will replace the deciduous molar is first seen starting to form after the deciduous root resorption begins, and it probably promotes additional resorption

    c. the deciduous tooth roots resorb rapidly and the tooth drops off the jaw, leaving the fully formed but uncalcified permanent tooth near the surface

    d. the deciduous tooth roots are slowly resorbed for a time; then for a brief period there is additional formation of cementum and adjacent bone, resulting in reattachment of the periodontal ligament fibers and a tightening of the tooth in the jaw; this is followed by root resorption; alternation of resorption and apposition takes place before the tooth finally loses its attachment in the mouth

104. The teeth of the permanent dentition undergo a slow movement known as *mesial drift*. This movement of a tooth is accompanied by a typical histologic picture in the bone supporting the tooth. For the present consideration, let us use as an example a mandibular second premolar which is undergoing mesial drift. If this tooth and its supporting bone structure were to be removed, sectioned in a mesiodistal plane, and studied with a microscope, there probably would be seen

    a. hisologic evidence of bone resorption in the trabecular bone apical to the tooth, and at the alveolar crest

    b. histologic evidence of bone resorption in the lamina dura (alveolar bone proper) on the distal side of the root, and bone apposition in the lamina dura on the mesial side of the root; the trabecular bone would show bone apposition

    c. histologic evidence of bone resorption in the lamina dura on the mesial side of the root, and bone apposition in the lamina dura on the distal side of the root; the trabecular bone would not be noticeably affected

    d. histologic evidence of bone resorption in the lamina dura on both the mesial and distal sides of the root, and bone apposition at the alveolar crest and at the root apex; the trabecular bone would not be noticeably altered

105. The position of the developing crown of the permanent maxillary third molar is

     a. posterior to the second maxillary molar with the occlusal surface directed slightly lingually

     b. in the maxillary tuberosity with the occlusal surface directed occlusally

     c. in the maxillary tuberosity with the occlusal surface directed somewhat distally and buccally

     d. posterior to the second maxillary molar rotated clockwise about 90 degrees

106. The position of the developing crown of the permanent mandibular third molar is

     a. a vertical position in the body of the mandible distal to the second molar

     b. in the ramus of the mandible, near the body, with the occlusal surface of the crown directed mesially

     c. in the body of the mandible, posterior to the second molar, with the occlusal surface directed distally

     d. in the ramus of the mandible with the occlusal surface directed upward

ANSWERS

1. a	20. c	39. d	58. a
2. d	21. b	40. c	59. b
3. c	22. d	41. d	60. c
4. a	23. c	42. a	61. c
5. d	24. c	43. b	62. d
6. b	25. c	44. d	63. c
7. d	26. a	45. a	64. a
8. b	27. d	46. d	65. c
9. c	28. d	47. c	66. c
10. a	29. b	48. b	67. d
11. b	30. b	49. c	68. b
12. c	31. b	50. d	69. c
13. d	32. c	51. a	70. b
14. a	33. d	52. b	71. c
15. c	34. d	53. a	72. d
16. a	35. c	54. b	73. d
17. b	36. c	55. c	74. c
18. b	37. b	56. b	75. b
19. d	38. b	57. d	76. a

77. b	85. d	93. d	101. b
78. a	86. d	94. d,c,c	102. c
79. d	87. b	95. b	103. d
80. b	88. c	96. b	104. c
81. a	89. a	97. c	105. c
82. c	90. c	98. d	106. b
83. c	91. b	99. c	
84. c	92. d	100. a	

REFERENCES

1. Bevelander, G.: *Essentials of Histology.* 6th Ed. St. Louis, The C. V. Mosby Co., 1967.
2. Permar, D.: *Oral Embryology and Microscopic Anatomy.* 4th Ed. Philadelphia, Lea & Febiger, 1967.

CHAPTER 2

PATHOLOGY

Elmer E. Kelln

1. Injury may best be defined as

    a. an alteration in the cells' homeostatic mechanism
    b. a cause of hemorrhage
    c. any trauma capable of causing pain
    d. that which will cause a temporary or lifelong disease

2. The primary function of the inflammatory process is

    a. to dilute the irritant
    b. to remove the irritant
    c. to remove the dead cells
    d. all of the above

3. The biologic and biochemical phenomenon of neutralizing, destroying, and removing an irritant with subsequent preparation of an injured area for repair is identified as

    a. regeneration
    b. infection
    c. metabolism
    d. inflammation

4. The cell which is probably responsible for the liberation of the agents that excite the early phases of the inflammatory process is the

    a. mast cell
    b. fibroblast
    c. melanocyte
    d. endothelial cell

5. When the phase of vascular dilatation occurs in the inflammatory process, the agent probably responsible for this single phenomenon is

    a. hyaluronidase
    b. histamine
    c. 5-hydroxytryptamine
    d. heparin

6. During the inflammatory phase of exudation, fluids leave the vascular bed. During the early minutes of this exudation, the fluid is primarily

    a. albumin and crystalloids
    b. colloids and globulins
    c. a serous transudate
    d. blood and fibrinogen

7. During the inflammatory phase of cellular exudation, the first cell to leave the vascular bed is the polymorphonuclear leukocyte. This cell is best recognized for the following function or property.

    a. opsinization and phagocytosis
    b. specific reaction with foreign proteins
    c. liberation of globulins and antibodies
    d. liberation of histamine and heparin

8. Pyogenic microorganisms have produced a suppurative exudate in an area. Drainage of this area causes a yellowish bloody fluid to escape. The best term for grossly describing this exudate is

    a. sanguinopurulent
    b. fibrinopurulent
    c. catarrhal
    d. serofibrinous

9. In an area of tissue repair, the formation of new endothelial cells that hollow out to allow a few blood cells to pass through them, and the association of these new vessels with new fibroblasts is termed

    a. granulomatous inflammation
    b. granulation tissue
    c. the phenomenon of exudation
    d. osteogenesis

10. When the defect caused by a knife wound fills in with coagulated blood elements, the first vital sign of repair is noted when

    a. endothelial cells invade clot
    b. fibroblasts invade clot
    c. the plasma cells migrate to area
    d. the collagen bundles form

11. Complete epithelialization over a tooth extraction socket is usually completed by the

    a. third day
    b. seventh day
    c. tenth day
    d. fourteenth day

12. A properly incised surgical wound has been sutured so that there is juxtaposition of the severed tissue surfaces. This wound is expected to heal by

    a. secondary intention
    b. the formation of a callus
    c. primary intention
    d. granulating tissue and subsequent healing from the base upward

13. When muscle is severed during a surgical procedure, the muscle will assume good normal function when anastomosis and healing has occurred. This is possible because

    a. muscle cells span the gap and join cut surfaces
    b. the two cut surfaces are joined by scar tissue
    c. each section functions regardless of the other
    d. the overlying skin and tissues produce desired movement

14. An individual experienced a fractured humerus and had the arm immobilized in a plaster cast for ten weeks. At the end of this period, the cast was removed and it was noted that the circumference of the arm in the biceps region had reduced by one cm. This reduction in size can be explained by which one of the following terms?

    a. hypertrophy
    b. nutritional atrophy
    c. disuse atrophy
    d. muscular dystrophy

15. The microscopic character of a scar on the cutaneous surface is described as

    a. dense collagenous tissue in which there are sclerosed capillaries and several sweat glands
    b. dense collagenous tissue with many sclerosed capillaries plus a few lymphocytes at the periphery
    c. loose fibrous tissue with many large capillaries and areas of blood pigment
    d. a calcified area in the dermis

16. During a postmortem examination the heart showed extensive evidence of fatty metamorphosis within the cardiac muscle. The most likely cause would be

    a. alcoholism and malnutrition
    b. hypertension and obesity
    c. obesity and overwork
    d. chemical poisoning in a rheumatic heart

17. The cells lining the proximal tubules in the kidney have taken up an excess of water, and microscopically appear distended, showing a pale granular cytoplasm. Into what category would this degeneration fall?

    a. fatty degeneration
    b. fat necrosis
    c. hyaline degeneration
    d. cloudy swelling

18. A person is known to have heart failure and consistent swelling of lower limbs. More specifically, this person has

    a. a fibrillating heart
    b. a heart block problem
    c. left sided heart failure
    d. right sided heart failure

19. An erythematous skin lesion would be seen in

    a. heavy x-ray exposure to the skin
    b. inflammation
    c. sunburn
    d. all of the above

20. A congested liver is a liver that is engorged with blood. Therefore, chronic passive congestion of the liver would be seen in

    a. left sided heart failure
    b. right sided heart failure
    c. left sided ventricular hypertrophy
    d. mitral stenosis

21. The rapid occlusion of the arterial blood supply will create an area of coagulation necrosis in that tissue dependent upon oxygenated blood. Such a lesion is known as

    a. an infarct
    b. congestion
    c. cellulitis
    d. an abscess

22. On final analysis, in order to have a thrombus form there must be

    a. a surplus of vitamin K in the blood
    b. a stasis in the flow of the blood
    c. a coagulase positive enzyme present
    d. injury to the endothelium

23. A thrombus is best defined as

    a. formation of a clot in the vessel of a deceased person
    b. formation of a clot within the vessel of a living person
    c. that which occurs when blood coagulates in a test tube
    d. that which only occurs in a coronary artery

24. In which of the following groups are all of the conditions capable of causing extensive enamel hypoplasia?

    a. pyrexia, increased fluorides, and congenital syphilis
    b. osteoporosis, diabetes, and fluorosis
    c. acquired syphilis, measles, and osteogenesis imperfecta
    d. acromegaly, hypoparathyroidism, and myxedema

25. In a developmental disease known as cleidocranial dystrophy, the individual has several edentulous areas; however, on roentgenographic examination the teeth are present but unerupted. Which of the following best defines this dental problem?

    a. false partial anodontia
    b. true partial anodontia
    c. false complete anodontia
    d. true complete anodontia

26. A patient presents himself with yellowish teeth and a lack of fully formed enamel. The diagnosis of amelogenesis imperfecta is made. Other physical findings are also noted on this person, the most likely of which are

    a. dwarfism, high arched palate, and cleft lip
    b. brittle bones, frontal bossing, and blue sclera
    c. blue eyes, lack of tearing, and blonde hair
    d. micrognathic mandible and ear defects

27. Should the maxillary process fail to unite with the globular process in the soft tissue as well as in the hard tissue derivatives, the result is

    a. a cleft anterior palate and lip
    b. a cleft lip and posterior palate
    c. a total cleft palate
    d. an oblique facial cleft

28. A biopsy of a base-of-the-tongue lesion in a 7-year-old female was reported as being made up of thyroid tissue. The probable reason for this report is that

    a. she has thyroid cancer and it has metastasized to the tongue
    b. the tongue has many heterotopic cells and these differentiated into glands and formed a thyroid tumor
    c. during embryogenesis the thyroid gland originates in the base of the tongue and in this case formed a lingual thyroid
    d. the mass was actually salivary glands and these were mistaken for thyroid tissues by the pathologist

29. The yellowish spots known as Fordyce's granules which are frequently observed on the cheek mucosa are actually

    a. ectopic sebaceous glands
    b. degenerated minor salivary glands
    c. islands of hyaline degeneration
    d. areas of lipomatoses in an obese person

30. The cleft between the embryonal branchial arches may entrap cells which cause future branchial cleft cysts. The location of such a cyst usually is on the

    a. side of the neck
    b. midline and anterior aspect of the neck
    c. back of the neck
    d. floor of the mouth

31. When the lingual embryonal processes fail to cover up the tuberculum impar, the resultant area seen on the dorsal surface of the tongue is termed

    a. geographic tongue
    b. rhomboid tongue
    c. bifid tongue
    d. uvula bifida

32. In congenital syphilis, the permanent incisors may represent Hutchinson's teeth; however, tooth malformation will not be present in primary teeth because

    a. primary teeth are resistant to spirochetal invasion
    b. the primary teeth will have already calcified by the time the spirochete infects the child
    c. the child becomes resistant from a blood transfusion
    d. in congenital syphilis, the mother becomes infected just before the child is born

33. A cyst is an epithelial lined cavity containing fluid. In a radicular cyst, the source of this epithelium is

    a. the primitive dental lamina
    b. multipotential cells in the apical region
    c. the endothelial cells of the pulp chamber
    d. the rests of Malassez in the periodontal ligament

34. The radicular cyst is so named because it is

    a. an independently arising lesion, unrelated to the periapical granuloma
    b. a common, but not inevitable, sequela of the periapical granuloma
    c. the inevitable sequela of the periapical granuloma at the root apex
    d. occasionally found on a vital tooth with a sound pulp

35. A 13-year-old girl has a large, tender, fluctuant mass in the midline of the hard palate and roentgenograms show a sharp punched-out radiolucency. Which of the following conditions is this most likely to be?

    a. torus palatinus
    b. median palatal cyst
    c. papillary cystadenoma
    d. adenoid cystic basal cell carcinoma

36. Primitive entrapped epithelial cells have formed a fissural cyst between the bony areas which embryonally represented the union of the globular and maxillary process. The exact location of this cyst is between the

    a. two maxillary incisors
    b. two mandibular incisors
    c. maxillary second premolar and first molar
    d. maxillary cuspid and lateral incisor

37. Sialolithiasis is a complication that may occur in any salivary gland duct; however, Wharton's duct is most frequently involved. The reason for this is

    a. Wharton's duct is the longest and most tortuous
    b. the submandibular gland is the lowest in anatomic position
    c. the tongue helps obstruct the flow of saliva
    d. the submandibular gland is weak and cannot express saliva

38. A salivary gland has been obstructed near its opening into the floor of the mouth. The gland has continued to produce saliva and has distended the duct, causing a large bluish bleb on the floor of the mouth which interferes with the tongue movements. This lesion is known as

    a. a ranula
    b. a phlegmon
    c. an aneurysm
    d. a parulis

39. Xerostomia is a term that means dry mouth. In one of the groups listed below all the conditions or diseases are associated with xerostomia. Identify the correct group.

    a. mixed tumors of the parotid and mumps
    b. extreme blood loss, puberty, and anemia
    c. anemia, Mikulicz's disease, and pregnancy
    d. diabetes, menopause, and radiation to salivary glands

40. The most common salivary gland tumor is the pleomorphic adenoma and the most common site for this tumor is in the

    a. minor salivary glands of the palate
    b. submental salivary glands
    c. parotid salivary glands
    d. submandibular salivary glands

41. An acute dento-alveolar abscess caused by streptococci is characterized by the fact that it

    a. always follows a pulpal exposure
    b. is completely walled off by a fibrous capsule
    c. is an accumulation of plasma cells and lymphocytes
    d. consists of a focus of neutrophilic infiltrate and early liquefaction degeneration

42. A 7-year-old girl presents a high fever. A few days prior the mother states that the girl had a sore throat and a cough. Upon examining the oral mucosa numerous red dots with white centers are noted. In all probability these oral lesions are

    a. Koplik's spots
    b. lichen planus striae
    c. herpetic lesions
    d. erythema multiforme lesions

43. Rheumatic fever may precipitate heart damage and mitral stenosis. The microorganism causing sensitization and subsequent heart damage is the

    a. group A Streptococcus
    b. Streptococcus viridans
    c. diplococcus
    d. group C Streptococcus

44. A patient presents an open lesion measuring 2 cm. on the buccal mucosa. The lesion is ulcerated, painless, and firm. The tuberculin tests were negative; serology positive. This lesion is a

    a. canker sore
    b. traumatic ulcer
    c. latent chancre
    d. pyogenic granuloma

45. The incidence of candidosis is most frequent in which one of the following combinations?

    a. childhood and middle age
    b. diabetes and childhood
    c. infants, diabetics, and aged females
    d. adolescence, pregnancy, and anemia

46. A circumscribed lesion containing intact and disintegrated polymorphonuclear neutrophils and surrounded by a fibrosed wall is known as

    a. cellulitis
    b. an abscess
    c. granulation tissue
    d. a fistula

47. Present observations reveal that acute ulcerative necrotizing gingivitis is

    a. purely an infection caused by oral bacilli and spirochetes
    b. a combination of infection, hypersensitivity, and constitutional problems
    c. a contagious disease seen mostly in soldiers
    d. a disease caused by lack of vitamin C

48. Phlegmonous inflammation is a diffuse inflammatory infectious disease characteristic of microorganisms capable of lysing the pyogenic membrane with fibrinolysin. Which group contains a causative microorganism and lytic enzyme?

    a. Staphylococcus and coagulase
    b. Mycobacterium tuberculosis and trypsin
    c. Borrelia vincenti and trypsin
    d. Streptococcus and streptokinase

49. Leukoplakia in itself means a white patch and has been a confusing term across the country. At present the term should be reserved for

    a. a premalignant lesion
    b. any white patch in the mouth
    c. cases of leukemia with oral manifestations
    d. cases of frank carcinoma

50. A skin disease has associated oral manifestations of white lines crossing each other forming lace-like patterns; the disease is

    a. psoriasis
    b. pemphigus
    c. lichen planus
    d. pityriasis rosea

51. A patient with pemphigus vulgaris, unless treated, would probably succumb to an infection because

    a. it is an infectious disease at onset
    b. it is a disease of the debilitated
    c. serum protein loss is high in this disease
    d. the open lesions become readily infected

52. Erythema multiforme's etiology in the past has been unknown; presently, it is considered to be related to a

    a. drug eruption
    b. mycotic infection
    c. collagen disease
    d. nutritional deficiency

53. A widening of the periodontal membrane to several times its normal width in a patient suffering from a systemic disease is probably based on

    a. severe edema as in hypothyroidism
    b. bone loss in osteoporosis
    c. collagen degeneration as in scleroderma
    d. traumatic occlusion as in tetanus

54. Upon a dental examination it was grossly noted that the teeth had a bluish appearance and roentgenographically noted that they lacked pulp chambers and had fine spindle-like roots. A further history revealed that this person has had numerous fractures since birth. One would suspect this to be a case of

    a. osteogenesis imperfecta with dentinogenesis imperfecta
    b. osteoporosis and ectodermal dysplasia
    c. amelogenesis imperfecta and osteopetrosis
    d. cleidocranial dysostosis

55. A syndrome comprising lack of development of the clavicle, under-development of the maxilla, over-retention of primary teeth, and delayed eruption of permanent teeth is known as

    a. Crouzon's disease
    b. Treacher-Collins syndrome
    c. Pierre Robin syndrome
    d. cleidocranial dysostosis

56. A completely edentulous patient comes to the dental office requesting the construction of a set of dentures. The dentist examines the roent-genogram of the patient's mouth before seeing the patient and con-cludes that all of the teeth have been extracted. When the dentist examines the patient, he notes that the patient has thin, sparse hair, dry skin, and malformed fingernails. History reveals that the patient has never had any natural teeth. The anodontia in this case is most probably associated with

    a. cleidocranial dysostosis
    b. ectodermal dysplasia
    c. hypothyroidism
    d. amelogenesis imperfecta

57. A set of oral roentgenograms revealed a loss of lamina dura, ground-glass bone, and lytic lesions in the jaws which proved to be giant cell tumors on microscopic examination. Which one of the following diseases does the patient have?

    a. acromegaly
    b. sickle cell anemia
    c. hypoparathyroidism
    d. hyperparathyroidism

58. A dark tan-like pigmentation is developing on pressure areas of the skin (such as under the belt line, wrist-watch band, etc). Orally a dark pigment is appearing on the prominent interdental papilla. Which disease would one suspect?

    a. diabetes
    b. adrenogenital syndrome
    c. kidney disease
    d. Addison's disease

59. A patient has been referred because of a nutritional problem. Find-ings show angular cheilosis, loss of filiform papilla, and a magenta tongue. This is a specific entity for which one of the following vitamin deficiencies?

    a. riboflavin
    b. thiamin
    c. nicotinic acid
    d. vitamin K

60. In scurvy there is an increase in capillary permeability resulting in free gingival bleeding. The vitamin that will correct this since it has a homeostatic effect on capillary permeability is

    a. vitamin A
    b. vitamin B
    c. vitamin C
    d. vitamin D

61. Which one of the following groups identifies a person who has hypothyroidism?

    a. high arched palate, large mandible, and glossodynia
    b. micrognathic mandible, large tongue, and hypertelorism
    c. myxedema of the tongue, slow eruption table, and poor root-to-crown ratio
    d. advanced size for age, precocious puberty, and early eruption table

62. Of all the blood dyscrasias, the one most often diagnosed by a dentist is acute leukemia. The gingival enlargement found in leukemia is due to

    a. an inflammatory infiltrate made up of leukemic cells
    b. the fluid exudate causing swelling
    c. fibroblastic proliferation
    d. inflammation because of poor oral hygiene

63. A person who has hypersecretion of hormones of the anterior pituitary as a child will become gigantic. If this phenomenon occurs after growth centers close, he has acromegaly. In acromegaly, certain bones increase in size; these are the

    a. maxilla, pelvic bone, and nasal bones
    b. mandible, frontal bone, hand bones, and foot bones
    c. mandible, humerus, and femur
    d. maxilla, radius, and ulna

64. An elderly male has an erythrocyte count of only one million. These cells are macrocytic and normochromic. He also has glossodynia and glossopyrosis. Which of the following blood diseases would he have?

    a. agranulocytosis
    b. polycythemia vera
    c. pernicious anemia
    d. leukemia

65. A person who has a persistent red blood cell count of 11,000,000 regardless of whether he lives at sea level or high in the Andes probably has

    a. anemia
    b. multiple myeloma
    c. leukemia
    d. polycythemia vera

66. The chief oral manifestation of agranulocytosis is

    a. deep necrotic ulcers
    b. a burning tongue
    c. a loss of the periodontal ligament
    d. swollen and hemorrhagic gingivae

67. The most common reason for finding melanotic mucosa in the oral cavity is

    a. racial
    b. that melanomas are frequent in the mouth
    c. Addison's disease
    d. Peutz-Jeghers disease

68. Green stain is a type of extrinsic stain found mainly on children's teeth and caused by chromogenic microorganisms. Which areas are mostly involved?

    a. gingival third of maxillary anterior teeth
    b. middle third of mandibular anterior teeth
    c. middle third of maxillary anterior teeth
    d. all teeth in the mouth with equal distribution

69. In a 3-year-old infant, all primary teeth show pigment picked up from bile obstruction. This obstruction must have occurred

    a. shortly after birth
    b. during early fetal life
    c. during late fetal life
    d. during the third year of life

70. A person has a single dark permanent central incisor. This discoloration could have been caused by any of the following *except*

    a. tetracycline intake
    b. trauma
    c. caries
    d. a restoration

71. A tooth turned dark because it was nonvital, a good example of
    a. an extrinsic stain
    b. an intrinsic stain
    c. amelogenesis imperfecta
    d. tetracycline stain

72. In this country, the most effective public health measure presently available as a deterrent to dental caries is
    a. the placing of vitamins in milk
    b. the straightening of malpositioned teeth
    c. topical application of fluorides
    d. fluoridating the water supplies

73. A mass that is loosely adherent to the tooth surface and is primarily made up of materia alba, microorganisms, and oral debris is known as
    a. dental caries
    b. a dental plaque
    c. calculus
    d. a protective film

74. A plaque on a tooth surface may have a pH of 6.9 which lowers to a pH value of 5.7 during mealtime. This lowering of pH is the result of
    a. eating citrus fruits during the meal
    b. acidogenic microorganisms fermenting carbohydrates
    c. acidosis created during a respiratory disease
    d. salivary glands producing saliva during meals

75. The process of dental caries formation is not fully understood; however, present day research does include at least three factors that must operate to produce caries. These are
    a. inheritance, diet, and race
    b. race, water supply, and action of microorganisms
    c. poor vitamin diet and action of proteolytic microorganisms on substrate
    d. action of microorganisms on diet in susceptible teeth

76. The pattern of tooth decalcification in pit and fissure caries has certain specific characteristics. Which of the following statements describes the pattern?
    a. The pattern is triangular with the base of the triangle toward the pulp.
    b. The pattern is triangular with the base of the triangle toward the tooth surface.
    c. The pattern is always ovoid in shape.
    d. The decalcification follows along enamel rods and the pattern shows a tubular destruction.

77. The manner in which fluoride suppresses dental caries is by

   a. making the enamel more resistant to acids
   b. blocking a bacterial enzyme and thereby inhibiting acid formation
   c. preventing microorganisms from deriving benefit from the breakdown process
   d. all of the above

78. Microscopically, the first degenerative sign noted in caries of the dentin is

   a. a fatty degeneration of the tubules
   b. the presence of bacteria in the tubules
   c. the formation of sclerotic dentin
   d. the disarrangement of odontoblasts

79. A male patient is 57 years old and has a gingivectomy. As a result, the root surfaces of several teeth are now grossly visible. The periodontist will plane the cementum off the root surface as a caries prevention process. In this case caries will be reduced

   a. because the underlying dentin has higher inorganic properties
   and therefore more caries resistance
   b. because the cementum has pores where Sharpey's fibers were
   attached and these are readily invaded by microorganisms
   c. because it is easier to cleanse debris from a smoother surface
   and thus oral hygiene is enhanced
   d. for all of the above reasons

80. Which one of the following statements is true?

   a. After the age of 35 years, more teeth are lost because of dental
   caries than for periodontal reasons.
   b. Periodontal disease is a disease of the aged and is unknown in
   children.
   c. The incidence of tooth loss in the fifth to seventh decade is
   shared equally by caries and by periodontal factors.
   d. After the age of 35 years, the chief cause of tooth loss is periodontal disease.

81. The depth at which the gingival sulcus can normally measure without eventually showing signs of inflammation is

   a. 1 to 3 millimeters
   b. 3 to 5 millimeters
   c. 5 to 7 millimeters
   d. under 10 millimeters

82. What percentage of the American population, aged over 40 years, have some form of inflammatory periodontal disease?

    a. 0 to 25%
    b. 25 to 50%
    c. 50 to 75%
    d. 75 to 90%

83. Should the degree of inflammation in a patient with periodontal involvement extend below the transseptal fibers, the term gingivitis should give way to the term

    a. periodontosis
    b. gingivosis
    c. periodontitis
    d. simple gingivitis

84. In a case of gingivitis the free and attached gingiva has a shiny gross appearance with loss of normal stippling. The histopathologic examination would show

    a. dense fibroblasts, lymphocytes, and neutrophils
    b. collagen bundles, plasma cells, and congestion
    c. mostly an inter- and intra-cellular edema
    d. passive congestion and granulation tissue

85. Present knowledge would indicate that chronic desquamative gingivitis (gingivosis) is a dystrophic disease affecting collagen bundles resulting from

    a. a sensitivity to a drug
    b. a vitamin deficient diet
    c. uncontrolled diabetes
    d. some hormonal disturbance

86. A patient suffers mental seizures and is placed on a Dilantin medication for control. Soon thereafter a periodontal problem results. Which of the following processes would you expect?

    a. a diffuse gingival hyperplasia
    b. atrophy of gingival tissue
    c. soft, spongy, edematous interdental papillae
    d. free bleeding from the gingival sulcus

87. A patient has presented himself to you with enlarged gingivae, free bleeding about the teeth, and halitosis. The person is given a routine prophylaxis and these three symptoms disappeared two days later when you again observed this patient. This dramatic response is based upon which of the following phenomena?

　　a. The removal of irritating factors during prophylaxis reduced the need for active hyperemia and inflammatory edema in the tissues.
　　b. A medication must have been given which reduced the swelling and hemorrhage.
　　c. The patient was given an antibiotic and this controlled the problem.
　　d. The patient must have had a circulatory or renal problem which is now corrected.

88. You have completed an office procedure for a dental prophylaxis. The future success of this treatment is primarily based upon the patient's

　　a. annual return visit and examination
　　b. diet during the next year
　　c. occupation and diet
　　d. carrying out of instructions in a home physiotherapy program

89. Carcinoma of the sinus may be of various histogenesis. Of the following, which group contain those one might expect?

　　a. osteogenic sarcoma, epidermoid carcinoma, and multiple myeloma
　　b. seminoma, cylindroma, lymphoepithelioma, and transitional cell carcinoma
　　c. transitional cell carcinoma, osteogenic sarcoma, epidermoid carcinoma, and lymphoepithelioma
　　d. osteogenic sarcoma, basal cell carcinoma, thymoma, and craniopharyngeoma

90. An oral lesion that has been diagnosed as a neurofibroma by a histologic section is apt to be associated with which of the following disease entities?

　　a. von Recklinghausen's disease
　　b. Weber's disease
　　c. Addison's disease
　　d. Sutton's disease

91. As a possible etiologic agent of oral carcinoma, which of the following tobacco habits is most closely related to oral cancer incidence?

    a. cigar smoking
    b. cigarette smoking
    c. pipe smoking
    d. tobacco chewing

92. Carcinoma of the buccal mucosa is most often preceded by

    a. heavy metal antisyphilitic therapy
    b. leukoplakia
    c. scar tissue
    d. ill-fitting dentures

93. Which of the following nodes would probably be involved with carcinoma of the left side of the lip near the angle?

    a. submental nodes
    b. deep cervical nodes
    c. submandibular nodes
    d. parotid nodes

94. Upon microscopic examination, a lesion is covered by stratified squamous epithelium, has underlying bundles of collagen fibers, occasional interspersed fibroblasts and blood vessels, but few inflammatory cells. Which of the following has been described?

    a. lipoma
    b. fibroma
    c. papilloma
    d. hemangioma

95. Of the following locations, the one in which epidermoid carcinoma has the least favorable prognosis is the

    a. lower lip
    b. hard palate
    c. buccal mucosa
    d. floor of the mouth

96. About 10% of all cancer occurs in the mouth. The most frequent histologic type of oral cancer is

    a. basal cell carcinoma
    b. adenocarcinoma
    c. squamous cell carcinoma
    d. endothelioma

97. Which of the following symptom complex groups describes osteo-genesis imperfecta?

    a. blue eyes, scanty hair, and oligodontia
    b. multiple osteomatosis, polyps in the large intestine, and desmoids
    c. elongation of bones of the hands and feet, and enlargement of the mandible
    d. blue sclera, brittle bones, and opalescent dentin

98. One of the following diseases has these hallmarks: obliteration of the auditory canal causing deafness, bony compression of the optic nerve causing blindness and a crowding of the marrow spaces resulting in anemia. The disease is

    a. osteomyelitis
    b. osteoporosis
    c. osteopetrosis
    d. Paget's disease

99. The firm, nodular tumor in the mid-line of the hard palate which is covered by normal appearing mucous membrane is most likely to be a

    a. squamous cell carcinoma
    b. giant cell tumor
    c. osteosarcoma
    d. torus palatinus

100. Cancer is the cause of 300,000 annual deaths in the United States. Presently as a cause of death it occupies

    a. first place
    b. second place
    c. third place
    d. fourth place

ANSWERS

1. a	12. c	23. b	34. b
2. d	13. b	24. a	35. b
3. d	14. c	25. a	36. d
4. a	15. b	26. c	37. a
5. c	16. a	27. a	38. a
6. c	17. d	28. c	39. d
7. a	18. d	29. a	40. c
8. a	19. d	30. a	41. d
9. b	20. b	31. b	42. a
10. a	21. a	32. b	43. a
11. d	22. d	33. d	44. c

45. c	59. a	73. b	87. a
46. b	60. c	74. b	88. d
47. b	61. c	75. d	89. c
48. d	62. a	76. a	90. a
49. a	63. b	77. d	91. c
50. c	64. c	78. a	92. b
51. c	65. d	79. d	93. c
52. a	66. a	80. d	94. b
53. c	67. a	81. a	95. d
54. a	68. a	82. d	96. c
55. d	69. b	83. c	97. d
56. b	70. a	84. c	98. c
57. d	71. b	85. d	99. d
58. d	72. d	86. a	100. b

REFERENCES

1. Anderson, W. A. D.: *Synopsis of Pathology.* 6th Ed. St. Louis, The C. V. Mosby Company, 1964, pp. 13–249.
2. Bhaskar, S. N.: *Synopsis of Oral Pathology.* 2nd Ed. St. Louis, The C. V. Mosby Company, 1965.
3. Kerr, D. A., and Ash, M. M.: *Oral Pathology.* 2nd Ed. Philadelphia, Lea & Febiger, 1965.
4. Manhold, J. H., and Bolden, T. E.: *Outline of Pathology.* Philadelphia, W. B. Saunders Company, 1960.
5. Shafer, W. G., Hine, M. K., and Levy, B. M.: *A Textbook of Oral Pathology.* 2nd Ed. Philadelphia, W. B. Saunders Co., 1963.
6. Steele, P. F.: *Dimensions of Dental Hygiene.* Philadelphia, Lea & Febiger, 1966, pp. 220–436.

CHAPTER 3

MICROBIOLOGY

Doris O. Powlen

1. The bacteria referred to as BCG are
   - a. pathogenic staphylococci
   - b. heat killed pneumococci
   - c. an attenuated strain of diphtheria
   - d. attenuated tubercle bacilli

2. Thermophilic bacteria grow best in an environment of
   - a. low pH
   - b. relatively high temperature
   - c. relatively high concentration of salt
   - d. reduced oxygen

3. A lytic strain of bacteria refers to one that
   - a. is autotrophic
   - b. is acid-fast
   - c. cannot survive in an environment of low pH
   - d. undergoes lysis owing to the influence of a bacteriophage

4. The incubation period of disease refers to the
   - a. generation time of a pathogenic organism
   - b. time required for the growth of a virulent culture in the laboratory
   - c. time required for an organism to complete a growth curve
   - d. period of time after the pathogenic organism enters the host until the symptoms of the disease are manifested

5. The arrangement of flagella in a tuft at one end of a bacterial cell is called
   - a. peritrichous
   - b. atrichous
   - c. lophotrichous
   - d. amphitrichous

6. Which of the following is *not* required to secure a maximal bacterial population?

    a. optimal temperature
    b. optimal pH
    c. sufficient light
    d. moisture

7. A group of filamentous organisms which occur in the dental plaque is

    a. Penicillium
    b. Neisseria
    c. Treponema
    d. Leptothrix

8. The cellular defense mechanism of the body refers to

    a. antibodies
    b. phagocytes
    c. enzymes
    d. mechanical barriers

9. When the symptoms of a disease are due to a toxemia, part of the immediate treatment would be the administration of

    a. a specific antitoxin
    b. a specific antigen
    c. gamma globulin
    d. antibiotics

10. The stage of a bacterial growth curve in which the death rate equals the reproduction rate is called the

    a. negative acceleration of growth phase
    b. accelerated death phase
    c. lag phase
    d. maximum stationary phase

11. The small nodular lesion produced in tuberculosis is called a

    a. fissure
    b. tubercle
    c. boil
    d. chancre

12. An endemic disease is one that

    a. spreads rapidly throughout a large population
    b. is noncommunicable
    c. occurs at a low but constant rate in a community
    d. has a long incubation period

13. The "clearance mechanism" refers to

    a. reducing the number of bacteria in the mouth by following a low carbohydrate diet

    b. reducing the number of bacteria in the mouth by such processes as eating, salivating, and movement of the lips, tongue, and cheeks

    c. removing debris from the mouth by brushing the teeth

    d. removing caries from the mouth by restoration treatment

14. Chemically, antibodies are

    a. carbohydrates

    b. lipids

    c. globulins

    d. enzymes

15. When stained by Gram's method, gram-positive organisms are colored

    a. purple

    b. red

    c. green

    d. brown

16. A leukocidin is a toxin that

    a. lyses red blood cells

    b. neutralizes leukocytes

    c. lyses white blood cells

    d. destroys connective tissue

17. Organisms that are able to derive their energy for growth and reproduction from simple inorganic substances are classified as

    a. autotrophic bacteria

    b. metatrophic bacteria

    c. heterotrophic bacteria

    d. anaerobic bacteria

18. A positive tuberculin test means that the patient

    a. is susceptible to tuberculosis

    b. has a hypersensitivity to the tubercle bacillus and/or its products

    c. is recovering from tuberculosis

    d. has an active case of tuberculosis

19. Bacteria receive their food, water, and oxygen and get rid of their waste products by the process of

    a. osmosis
    b. plasmoptysis
    c. fission
    d. hydrolysis

20. Fluoridation of water supplies may interfere with caries increment in children who drink the water by

    a. inhibiting acid production of bacteria
    b. inhibiting growth of bacteria
    c. combining with enamel and dentin and thus lowering the solubility of these substances in acid
    d. destroying enzyme constituents in the bacteria cell

21. The man who developed the smallpox vaccine was

    a. Pasteur
    b. Jenner
    c. Koch
    d. van Leeuwenhoek

22. When two organisms growing together can produce a reaction which neither can produce alone, the relationship is termed

    a. synergism
    b. mutualism
    c. symbiosis
    d. commensalism

23. Because of faulty sterilization of syringes in the dental office, which of the following viral diseases has been transmitted to patients?

    a. mumps
    b. serum hepatitis
    c. influenza
    d. trench mouth

24. The most poisonous bacterial toxin known to man is produced by the organism

    a. Pseudomonas aeruginosa
    b. Pasteurella tularensis
    c. Brucella abortus
    d. Clostridium botulinum

25. Bacteria reproduce by the process of

    a. binary fission
    b. budding
    c. germination
    d. sporulation

26. Dental cavities begin at discrete localized spots on the surfaces of the tooth. This localization is due to the formation of

    a. antibodies
    b. dental plaques
    c. hyaluronidase
    d. lysozyme

27. An antibacterial solution which inhibits the reproduction of an organism, but does not kill it, is said to be

    a. chemoprophylactic
    b. bacteriocidal
    c. hemolytic
    d. bacteriostatic

28. That part of a bacterial cell which helps to provide resistance to phagocytosis is the

    a. nucleus
    b. capsule
    c. spore
    d. cell wall

29. When an immune host comes in contact with a pathogenic organism for the second time, there is often a rapid increase in concentration of the antibody level in the serum. This reaction is called

    a. plasmolysis
    b. the opsonic reaction
    c. anaphylaxis
    d. anamnestic reaction

30. The Embden-Meyerhof scheme explains the

    a. microbial breakdown of proteins
    b. microbial breakdown of fats
    c. aerobic breakdown of carbohydrates
    d. anaerobic breakdown of carbohydrates

31. Bacteremia refers to

    a. the presence of bacteria in the blood
    b. the inhibition of bacteria
    c. the death of bacteria via lysis
    d. pus in the blood

32. The earliest oral flora of the newborn develops from

   a. contamination by air
   b. contact with persons first handling the child
   c. passage through the birth canal
   d. the first food ingested

33. The arrangement of bacilli in parallel lines is called

   a. streptobacilli grouping
   b. palisade grouping
   c. microbacilli grouping
   d. sarcina grouping

34. Koch's postulate must be followed in order to prove the

   a. identity of an unknown organism
   b. fermentation pattern of an organism
   c. etiology of an infection
   d. proper treatment of a disease

35. An arthropod that aids in the transmission of disease is called a

   a. fomite
   b. vector
   c. carrier
   d. host

36. A specific amount of sodium chloride is added to a culture medium in order to maintain an optimum osmotic pressure for the organisms. This medium would be called

   a. isotonic
   b. hypertonic
   c. hydrotonic
   d. hypotonic

37. Which one of the following characteristics is *not* true of a mutation?

   a. It is an inherited trait.
   b. It arises suddenly rather than insidiously.
   c. It is usually most beneficial to the organisms.
   d. It is a genetic change.

38. Organisms described as being filterable, submicroscopic, and obligate parasitic are

   a. viruses
   b. bacteria
   c. fungi
   d. spirochetes

39. Organisms that grow best in an acid environment are called
    a. acidophilic
    b. aciduric
    c. basophilic
    d. acidogenic

40. The streptococcal organisms that produce a green zone around a colony on blood agar are called
    a. alpha hemolytic
    b. gamma hemolytic
    c. indifferent
    d. beta hemolytic

41. The "Schick test" determines susceptibility to
    a. tuberculosis
    b. botulism
    c. diphtheria
    d. scarlet fever

42. Combining cellular antigen with its specific antibody plus complement in proper proportions (under proper conditions) results in
    a. lysis of the antigen
    b. formation of a toxoid
    c. production of an autogenous vaccine
    d. increased concentration of the antibody

43. A sporangium is a
    a. free spore
    b. fungus
    c. bacterial cell that contains an endospore
    d. virus that infects the oral cavity

44. Viruses are cultivated in the laboratory by use of a technique known as
    a. tissue culture
    b. centrifugation
    c. tissue transformation
    d. electrophoresis

45. The process whereby a free spore develops into a vegetative cell is called
    a. vegetation
    b. transduction
    c. sporulation
    d. germination

46. The temperature that would produce the shortest generation time for an organism is the
    a. minimum temperature
    b. thermal death point
    c. optimum temperature
    d. maximum temperature

47. Subacute bacterial endocarditis is an infection of the
    a. intestines
    b. lungs
    c. kidney
    d. heart valves

48. The enzyme produced by pathogenic staphylococci whose action results in the clotting of blood plasma is called
    a. streptodornase
    b. coagulase
    c. hyaluronidase
    d. catalase

49. Cholera is an infection of the
    a. intestinal tract   lower
    b. urinary tract
    c. respiratory tract
    d. liver

50. The most abundant organic compound found in a bacterial cell is
    depends on bacteria
    a. lipid
    b. carbohydrate
    c. protein
    d. water

51. Vincent's infection is associated with an increase in number of which of the following organisms commonly found in the mouth?
    a. Borrelia vincenti and Fusiformis dentium
    b. Diplococcus pneumoniae and Alcaligenes faecalis
    c. Staphylococcus aureus and Streptococcus salivarius
    d. Lactobacillus casei and Escherichia coli

52. Microscopic single celled plants that do not contain chlorophyl, and reproduce by transverse binary fission are known as
    a. molds
    b. yeast
    c. protozoa
    d. bacteria

53. An antibiotic is

    a. a component of gamma globulin which protects the host against pathogenic organisms

    b. synonymous with antibody

    c. a biological product which inhibits or kills other microorganisms

    d. a cellular defense mechanism

54. Which of the following reactions is associated with the sensitivity of bacteria to various antibiotics?

    a. fermentation

    b. pigment production

    c. Gram reaction

    d. action in gelatin

55. The acid-fast stain is useful in the diagnosis of

    a. diphtheria

    b. pneumonia

    c. Vincent's infection trench   mouth

    d. tuberculosis

56. The oral manifestation most commonly observed in primary syphilis is

    a. the appearance of white patches on the tongue

    b. a fever blister on the lip

    c. an increase in the lactobacilli in the oral flora

    d. the formation of an ulcer on the lip

57. An infection that originates at one area of the body but spreads to and localizes in other parts of the body is called a

    a. local infection

    b. generalized infection

    c. chronic infection

    d. focal infection

58. The organism that produces food poisoning owing to its production of "enterotoxin" is a member of the genus

    a. Salmonella

    b. Shigella

    c. Staphylococcus

    d. Clostridium

59. The grouping of the different types of bacterial cells is largely influenced by the

    a. generation time

    b. post fission movements

    c. presence of spores

    d. cytoplasmic membrane

60. The first step in the identification of an unknown culture is to

    a. do an acid-fast stain
    b. do a dark-field examination
    c. determine its motility
    d. isolate it in pure culture

61. The aerobic bacteria that occur in the greatest numbers in the oral flora are the

    a. fusiforms
    b. yeast
    c. lactobacilli
    d. streptococci

62. Simple staining of bacteria can give us the following information.

    a. chemical nature of the cell
    b. acid-fastness of the organism
    c. size, shape, and grouping of the bacteria
    d. presence of a capsule

63. Media that will support growth of most kinds of bacteria are called

    a. differential media
    b. complete media
    c. natural media
    d. selective media

64. A change in the colony morphology of an organism is known as

    a. dissociation
    b. transduction
    c. mutation
    d. induction

65. The hanging drop method of examining bacteria is used mainly to observe

    a. motility
    b. Gram reaction
    c. size of organism
    d. spirochetes

66. Artificial active immunity may be obtained by introduction into the host of

    a. antiserum
    b. antitoxin
    c. opsonins
    d. heat killed bacteria

67. Which of the following does *not* influence the occurrence of infection in man?

    a. virulence of the organism
    b. site of entrance of the organism
    c. amount of complement in the host's serum
    d. number of organisms infecting the host

68. An organic catalyst produced by a living cell is known as an

    a. enzyme
    b. antibody
    c. agglutinin
    d. endotoxin

69. The "Quellung" reaction is important in the identification of

    a. pneumococci
    b. spirochetes
    c. enteric organisms
    d. streptococci

70. The exchange of genetic material from one cell to another by means of a phage carrier is known as

    a. transformation
    b. recombination
    c. transduction
    d. dissociation

71. When two organisms must live together for survival, the relationship is called

    a. antibiosis
    b. symbiosis
    c. mutualism
    d. commensalism

72. Which of the following represents the bacteriologic breakdown sequence of proteins?

    a. proteins⟷polypeptides⟷amino acids⟷peptones
    b. proteins⟷peptide⟷peptone⟷amino acids
    c. proteins⟷peptones⟷polypeptides⟷peptides⟷amino acids
    d. proteins⟷peptones⟷peptides⟷polypeptide⟷amino acids

73. Bacteria that live on dead organic material are called

    a. autotrophic organisms
    b. pathogenic organisms
    c. saprophytic organisms
    d. paratrophic organisms

74. The clumping reaction observed when a cellular antigen is brought into contact with its homologous antibody (under proper conditions) is called

    a. lysis
    b. phagocytosis
    c. agglutination
    d. precipitation

75. An antibody which specifically embraces phagocytosis is called

    a. a serum
    b. an opsonin
    c. a precipitin
    d. an agglutinogen

76. Intermittent sterilization is carried out in the

    a. hot air ovens
    b. autoclave
    c. Arnold sterilizer
    d. incubator

77. For life, obligate aerobes require

    a. a living host
    b. an oxygen free environment
    c. organic carbon and nitrogen
    d. molecular oxygen

78. The autoclave is one of the most effective means of sterilizing media and equipment because it employs

    a. dry heat at high temperatures
    b. low pressure
    c. moist heat at high temperature
    d. sonic vibrations

79. Spores benefit a bacterial cell because they provide the organism with

    a. motility
    b. resistance to adverse conditions
    c. pathogenicity
    d. acid-fastness

80. Which of the following is *not* effective as a means of sterilization?

    a. hot air oven
    b. ultraviolet rays
    c. autoclave
    d. incubator

81. A dentist should give prophylactic antibiotic treatment if the patient has a history of

     a. kidney damage
     b. tuberculosis
     c. rheumatic fever
     d. syphilis

82. An example of a local skin allergy is

     a. serum sickness
     b. anaphylaxis
     c. hay fever
     d. the Arthus reaction

83. A naturally occurring mutation is called

     a. an induced mutation
     b. a selective mutation
     c. an adaptation
     d. a spontaneous mutation

84. Organisms which require an environment free of molecular oxygen are called

     a. anaerobes
     b. autotrophs
     c. aerobes
     d. heterotrophs

85. Most pathogenic organisms can be classified as

     a. psychrophilic
     b. acidogenic
     c. mesophilic
     d. autotrophic

86. A "spreading factor" produced by pneumococci and streptococci is a metabolic product called

     a. antitoxin
     b. precipitin
     c. hyaluronidase
     d. streptokinase

87. An attenuated organism is one that is

     a. heat killed
     b. a nonpathogenic mutant of a previous pathogenic organism
     c. a toxin producer
     d. isolated from the host and then reinjected in a nonliving state

88. The presence of acid-fast organisms in the sputum suggests that the patient has

    a. pneumonia
    b. tuberculosis
    c. whooping cough
    d. pneumonic plague

89. The bacteriocidal action of sunlight is mainly due to

    a. infrared radiation
    b. x-rays
    c. ultraviolet radiation
    d. beta rays

90. Most upper respiratory infections are spread via

    a. fomites
    b. food
    c. water
    d. air

91. Which of the following exemplifies a mixed infection?

    a. Herpes simplex
    b. Typhoid fever
    c. Vincent's infection
    d. Tuberculosis

92. Susceptibility to caries may be indicated if the saliva contains a high concentration of

    a. Bacillus subtilis
    b. Staphylococcus aureus
    c. Lactobacillus casei
    d. Escherichia coli

93. The temperature that destroys all bacteria in a given culture within 10 minutes is known as

    a. optimum temperature
    b. thermoduric temperature
    c. maximum temperature
    d. thermal death point

94. A poisonous substance released from a bacterial cell upon the lysis
of the cell is called

    a. a toxoid
    b. an endotoxin
    c. toxemia
    d. mitochondria

95. A heat labile reagent required for bacterial or cell lysis is

    a. a complement
    b. an agglutination
    c. a lysinogen
    d. a hemolysin

96. The stimuli that call for the production of protective mechanisms
in the body are called

    a. antibodies
    b. hemolysins
    c. complement
    d. antigens

97. Endospores are formed by members of the genus

    a. Micrococcus
    b. Streptococcus
    c. Bacillus
    d. Escherichia

98. The foreign substances that cause hypersensitive reactions in a host
are called

    a. reagins
    b. antibodies
    c. allergens
    d. opsonins

99. The "Schultz-Charlton reaction" is diagnostic for

    a. diphtheria
    b. serum hepatitis
    c. scarlet fever
    d. typhoid fever

100. A haptene functions as a

    a. partial antigen
    b. reagin
    c. partial antibody
    d. complete antigen

ANSWERS

1. d	26. b	51. a	76. c
2. b	27. d	52. d	77. d.
3. d	28. b	53. c	78. c
4. d	29. d	54. c	79. b
5. c	30. d	55. d	80. d.
6. c	31. a	56. d	81. c
7. d	32. c	57. d	82. d
8. b	33. b	58. c	83. d
9. a	34. c	59. b	84. a
10. d	35. b	60. d	85. c
11. b	36. a	61. d	86. c
12. c	37. c	62. c	87. b
13. b	38. a	63. b	88. b
14. c	39. a	64. a	89. c
15. a	40. a	65. a	90. d
16. c	41. c	66. d	91. c
17. a	42. a	67. c	92. c
18. b	43. c	68. a	93. d
19. a	44. a	69. a	94. b
20. c	45. d	70. c	95. a
21. b	46. c	71. b	96. d
22. a	47. d	72. c	97. c
23. b	48. b	73. c	98. c
24. d	49. a	74. c	99. c
25. a	50. c	75. b	100. a

REFERENCES

1. Burnet, G. W., and Scherp, H. W.: *Oral Microbiology and Infectious Diseases.* 2nd Ed. Baltimore, Williams & Wilkins Co., 1962.
2. Frobisher, M.: *Fundamentals of Microbiology.* 7th Ed. Philadelphia, W. B. Saunders Co., 1962.
3. Lamanna, C., and Mallette, M. F.: *Basic Bacteriology.* 3rd Ed. Baltimore, Williams & Wilkins Co., 1965.
4. Smith, D. T., Conant, N. F., and Oberman, J. F.: *Zinsser Microbiology.* 13th Ed. New York, Appleton-Century-Croft, 1964.

CHAPTER 4

PHYSIOLOGY

Carroll G. Bennett

1. Nerve cells may be classified according to the number of cytoplasmic processes extending from the cell body. The most common type found in the human nervous system is

   a. nonpolar
   b. unipolar
   c. multipolar
   d. semipolar

2. Many of the cranial and spinal nerve processes are invested by a layer of material called myelin. The general chemical nature of this material is

   a. carbohydrate
   b. lipid
   c. steroid
   d. protein

3. End organs for pressure, temperature, and pain are distributed in the skin as exteroceptors. Specialized end organs which respond to cold are known as

   a. brushes of Ruffini
   b. nodes of Ranvier
   c. end bulbs of Krause
   d. Meissner's corpuscles

4. Nervous tissue consists of conducting units called neurons and supporting units called neuroglial cells. The function of the neuron processes known as dendrites is

   a. relaying impulses to the cell body
   b. transmitting impulses away from the cell body
   c. integrating impulses within the cell body
   d. conducting impulses to axons which transmit them into the cell body

5. The membrane covering which appears to be responsible for the regenerative ability of peripheral nerve fibers is called the

   a. myelin
   b. soma
   c. axoplasm
   d. neurilemma

6. Nerve tissue responds to a number of different types of stimuli provided the stimuli is of sufficient strength and duration. When the energy of an applied stimulus is too low to bring about initiation of a nerve impulse the stimulus is said to be

   a. at threshold
   b. supramaximal
   c. subliminal
   d. subrefractory

7. Nervous tissue that has been stimulated, has responded, and is now in the initial phase of the absolute refractory period

   a. will respond to a subliminal stimulus
   b. will respond to a threshold stimulus
   c. will respond to a supramaximal stimulus
   d. is no longer excitable and will not respond

8. The electrical potential (voltage) difference between the inside and the outside of the cell membrane is known as the

   a. membrane potential
   b. potential difference
   c. refractory potential
   d. intracellular potential gradient

9. Electrical potentials are dependent upon the effectiveness of the cell membrane in

   a. prohibiting the flow of K^+ ions
   b. separating the interstitial fluid from the intracellular cytoplasm
   c. allowing the free passage of Na^+ ions
   d. prohibiting the flow of Cl^- ions

10. Two of the most important ions involved in the cellular membrane potential are Na^+ and Cl^-. These ions are distributed

    a. primarily inside the cell
    b. approximately equally on both sides of the cell membrane
    c. primarily outside the cell
    d. with most of the Na^+ inside the cell and most of the Cl^- outside the cell

11. The K^+ ion concentration is higher within the cell than it is outside the cell. The magnitude of this difference of K^+ ion concentration within the cell is about

    a. 2 times higher than on the outside
    b. 10 times higher than on the outside
    c. 30 times higher than on the outside
    d. 80 times higher than on the outside

12. Single nerve and muscle fibers respond to a threshold stimulus by

    a. full conduction of the impulse and full contraction of the muscle fiber regardless of the strength of the stimulus
    b. slow conduction of the impulse and partial contraction of the muscle fiber when stimulated by weak stimuli
    c. rapid conduction of the impulse and maximal contraction of the muscle fiber when stimulated by strong stimuli
    d. a response identical to the manner that nerves and muscles (groups of fibers) exhibit

13. The velocity of a nerve impulse is dependent on factors such as the

    a. strength of the stimulus
    b. size, type, and physiologic condition of the nerve fiber
    c. duration of the stimulus
    d. type of stimulation applied to the nerve fiber

14. Nerve fibers which show the highest impulse velocity are

    a. large myelinated nerves
    b. small myelinated nerves
    c. large unmyelinated nerves
    d. small unmyelinated nerves

15. During the active phase of impulse conduction of a nerve fiber, one would find

    a. an increase in oxygen consumption and heat production
    b. a decrease in oxygen consumption and heat production
    c. an increase in oyxgen consumption and decrease in heat production
    d. a decrease in oygen consumption and increase in heat production

16. The first step in the initiation of a spike potential of nerve fibers is

    a. a closing of "sodium gates" thereby keeping Na^+ outside the axon
    b. a rapid outflow of K^+ ions
    c. a decrease in cell membrane permeability allowing Na^+ ions to enter the axon
    d. a leaking of Cl^- ions which neutralize available Na^+ ions

17. One of the accelerating forces which influence the movement of ions through a cell membrane is

    a. attraction of unlike charges in the same region
    b. repulsion between like charges
    c. migration of ions due to thermal agitation
    d. viscous resistance to motion of the ions

18. The characteristic activities of protoplasm are

    A. metabolism
    B. excretion
    C. respiration
    D. digestion

    a. all of the above
    b. only A, C, and D
    c. only B, C, and D
    d. only A, B, and C

19. Various parts of each cell have specific functions. One of the functions of the nucleus is

    a. cellular metabolism
    b. regeneration of injured cells
    c. synthesis of new protein
    d. secretory activities

20. The property of protoplasm which enables it to react to sudden changes in the environment is

    a. contractility
    b. elasticity
    c. irritability
    d. conductivity

21. When an external stimulus is applied to a muscle, after a short interval the muscle begins to contract. This short interval between stimulation and contraction is the

    a. refractory period
    b. latent period
    c. irritability period
    d. subconductive period

22. Cardiac muscle differs from skeletal muscle in several ways. One important difference is that cardiac muscle

    a. follows a pattern of graded response to graded stimulus
    b. requires a longer treppe period
    c. obeys the all-or-none law
    d. contractions increase as more motor units are involved

23. Incomplete tetanus results when rapid stimuli are repeatedly applied to a muscle and only partial relaxation is permitted. The term applied to this incompleted tetanus is

    a. clonus
    b. treppe
    c. isotonic contracture
    d. isometric contracture

24. Single subthreshold stimuli applied to a muscle will not cause a contraction. However, if these subliminal stimuli are repeated rapidly the muscle responds. This effect results from

    a. an additive effect of the stimuli
    b. a change in the membrane potential at the motor end plate of the muscle fiber
    c. an alteration of the length of intermuscle fibers
    d. an alteration of the treppe refractory period of the muscle fibers

25. Complete tetanus results when rapid stimulation causes a smooth fusion of contractions. This phenomenon is possible in

    A. cardiac muscle
    B. smooth muscle
    C. skeletal muscle

    a. only A and B
    b. only B and C
    c. only C
    d. only A

26. Electrical impulses carried by axons to skeletal muscles are transmitted to the underlying membranes by the liberation of a special material at the neuromuscular junction. This special material is

    a. adenosinetriphosphate
    b. creatine phosphate
    c. lactic acid
    d. acetylcholine

27. Heat given off during muscle activity is divided into initial heat, produced during contraction, and delayed heat, produced during the recovery period. One difference between these types of heat is that

    a. the delayed heat is produced more slowly
    b. the initial heat is produced more slowly
    c. considerably more delayed heat is produced
    d. considerably more initial heat is produced

28. Initial muscle contractions occur in the absence of oxygen. Repeated contraction results in the disappearance of

    a. adenosinediphosphate
    b. creatine phosphate
    c. glycogen
    d. acetylcholine

29. The contraction of muscle fibers requires a source of energy. The initial supply of energy is released when

    a. phosphate is split from adenosinetriphosphate
    b. phosphate is combined with adenosinetriphosphate
    c. glucose phosphate is split from glycogen
    d. phosphate is combined with glycogen forming glucose phosphate

30. The arithmetic difference between systolic and diastolic pressure is called the

    a. arterial pressure
    b. pulse pressure
    c. blood pressure
    d. capillary pressure

31. Blood is forced in a pulsating manner through the arteries by the pumping action of the cardiac muscle. By the time blood reaches the capillary bed it

    a. exhibits a continuous flow as in veins
    b. maintains a pulsatile flow as in arteries
    c. is under no pressure
    d. is under maximum pressure as a result of the small diameter of the vessel

32. Clinically, blood pressure in man is measured by a

    a. mercury manometer
    b. sphygmomanometer
    c. strain gauge manometer
    d. aneroid manometer

33. The normal blood pressure for a healthy young adult (20 to 25 years old) is

    a. 120 mm. of mercury systolic, 80 mm. of mercury diastolic
    b. 80 mm. of mercury systolic, 120 mm. of mercury diastolic
    c. 180 mm. of mercury systolic, 110 mm. of mercury diastolic
    d. 90 mm. of mercury systolic, 150 mm. of mercury diastolic

34. The growth of the embryo is dependent upon nutrition, which is supplied through the placenta. Oxygenated blood from the placenta is carried to the embryo by the

    a. umbilical arteries
    b. ductus venosus
    c. umbilical veins
    d. ductus arteriosus

35. In determining blood types the contents of both erythrocytes and plasma are important. One of the determining factors contained in erythrocytes is

    a. agglutinins
    b. agglutinogens
    c. antibodies
    d. erythroglutinins

36. The serologic blood type which can be donated to individuals of any other blood group is

    a. AB
    b. A
    c. B
    d. O

37. If the heart of a resting man is pumping 70 ml. of blood per minute and his heart rate is 60 per minute, the cardiac output is

    a. 42 liters
    b. 4.2 liters
    c. 84 liters
    d. 8.4 liters

38. Physiologically, the heart functions as two pumps, one forcing blood through the pulmonary circulation and the other forcing blood through the systemic circulation. The compartment with the heaviest muscular walls is the

    a. left atrium
    b. left ventricle
    c. right atrium
    d. right ventricle

39. In the human heart, a small mass of specialized tissue located in the right atrium serves as the pacemaker for cardiac contractions and is known as the

    a. atrioventricular node
    b. Purkinje fibers
    c. sinu-atrial node
    d. atrioventricular bundle

40. When the human heart is beating at a rate of 70 per minute, the duration of one complete cardiac cycle is about 0.8 second. This cycle is divided into four phases. The phase which lasts the shortest period of time is the

    a. atrial systole
    b. atrial diastole
    c. ventricular systole
    d. ventricular diastole

41. Respiration involves gaseous exchange at two sites, one across the respiratory membrane with the blood of the pulmonary circulation and the other between the systemic capillaries and the cells. The exchange between the respiratory membrane and the pulmonary circulation is known as

    a. anoxic respiration
    b. hypoxic respiration
    c. internal respiration
    d. external respiration

42. If man, during a period of work, receives a deficient supply of oxygen accompanied by an excessive increase in carbon dioxide in the body, the condition is known as

    a. hypoxia
    b. anoxia
    c. asphyxia
    d. carboxia

43. During the respiratory phase of inspiration, air enters the lungs and descends into the deeper structure as a result of

    a. an increase in the intrapulmonic pressure
    b. a decrease in the intrapulmonic pressure
    c. an increase in atmospheric pressure
    d. a decrease in atmospheric pressure

44. The maximum volume of air that can be exchanged in a single respiratory cycle is called the

    a. residual capacity
    b. vital capacity
    c. tidal capacity
    d. complemental capacity

45. The volume of air that is inspired and expired by a person who is resting and breathing quietly is called the

    a. tidal air
    b. vital air
    c. supplemental air
    d. complemental air

46. Activity of a person regulates the type of respiration. Normal quiet breathing is known as

    a. dyspnea
    b. apnea
    c. eupnea
    d. tachypnea

47. During quiet breathing about 500 ml. of air is inspired. Considering the dead space and total lung volume, what percentage of air is renewed in a quiet respiratory cycle?

    a. 10 to 15%
    b. 30 to 35%
    c. 50 to 55%
    d. 70 to 75%

48. Oxyhemoglobin formation in arterial blood at the alveoli exchange level is favored by

    a. high nitrogen partial pressure
    b. low oxygen partial pressure
    c. high carbon dioxide pressure
    d. low carbon dioxide pressure

49. Respiration is controlled by the respiratory centers in the

    a. spinal cord
    b. medulla
    c. cerebrum
    d. thalamus

50. Anoxia results when the oxygen supply is inadequate to meet the oxygen requirements of the body. When the deficiency of oxygen results from inadequate transport (i.e., circulatory failure) the condition is called

    a. stagnant anoxia
    b. anoxic anoxia
    c. histotoxic anoxia
    d. anemia anoxia

51. Enzymes are substances produced by cells that act as catalysts. They are named according to their action, thus a starch-splinting enzyme would be called

   a. lipase
   b. amylase
   c. protease
   d. proteinase

52. The first step in digestion begins in the oral cavity. The most important function of saliva is to

   a. make the food more alkaline
   b. change starch to maltose
   c. dissolve the solid substances bringing them in contact with taste buds
   d. change starch to glucose

53. The major acid found in gastric juices of the stomach is

   a. acetic acid
   b. lactic acid
   c. sulfuric acid
   d. hydrochloric acid

54. The first step in gastric digestion is the action of the gastric acid upon

   a. protein
   b. starch
   c. fat
   d. carbohydrate

55. Salivary secretions are stimulated involuntarily through excitation of nerve endings in the mouth. The type of secretions vary with the stimuli. Moist foods and large particles bring about a

   a. copious, watery secretion
   b. scant, sticky secretion
   c. decreased amount of thin saliva
   d. copious, ropy secretion

56. There are 3 phases involved in the secretion of gastric juice, the cephalic phase, the gastric phase, and the intestinal phase. The gastric phase is initiated by the

   a. presence of food in the mouth
   b. presence of fat in the intestine
   c. distention of the pylorus
   d. secretion of saliva

57. The release of pancreatic secretions results from both hormonal stimulation and nervous system control. The secretion resulting from hormonal stimulation contains

    a. trypsin
    b. trypsinogen
    c. secretin
    d. cholecystokinin

58. Two types of movement are found in the small intestine, one carries the chyme onward while the other churns and mixes the chyme with the digestive juices. The type of movement that mixes and churns the chyme is known as

    a. rhythmical segmentation
    b. peristaltic waves
    c. circulo-muscular relaxation
    d. pyloric sphincter contration

59. One important constituent of gastric juice is pepsin, which functions chiefly in the

    a. digestion of fats
    b. hydrolysis of starch
    c. initial breakdown of proteins
    d. digestion of carbohydrates

60. The relation between the volume of oxygen used and the amount of carbon dioxide formed is called the respiratory quotient. This calculation is useful in indicating the type of food being burned. A respiratory quotient of 1 would indicate a diet consisting chiefly of

    a. fat
    b. protein
    c. carbohydrates
    d. mixed fat and protein

61. A major component of urine is water. In a normal 24 hour period, water makes up what percentage of the total urine volume?

    a. 20%
    b. 50%
    c. 75%
    d. 95%

62. The first step in the formation of urine occurs in

    a. Bowman's capsule
    b. the glomeruli
    c. the proximal tubules
    d. Henle's loop

63. One important function of the kidneys is the regulation of acid-base balance in the blood. Adjustment of pH occurs mainly in
   a. the glomeruli
   b. the distal tubules
   c. the proximal tubules
   d. Henle's loop

64. In an average man the entire blood volume passes through the kidneys about
   a. three times per hour
   b. five times per hour
   c. ten times per hour
   d. fifteen times per hour

65. Normal body temperature represents a range rather than a single value. When the body temperature falls below normal (37°C.) internal heat is produced by
   a. sweating and panting
   b. unconscious tensing of muscles
   c. increased skin circulation
   d. liberation of carbon dioxide into lungs

66. Body temperature is regulated by temperature-sensitive nuclei of the hypothalamus. The "thermostatic" neurons respond to
   a. blood temperature
   b. skin temperature
   c. oxygen-carbon dioxide lung ratio
   d. external temperature of the head and neck region

67. Fever accompanying bacterial disease and infection is caused by
   a. bacterial attack on the hypothalamus
   b. pyogenic material released from injured cells
   c. presence of pathogenic organisms in the blood
   d. alteration of carbon dioxide content in the lungs

68. The formation of tissue fluid is related to the ratio between the filtration pressure and the protein osmotic pressure of the blood in the capillaries. Tissue fluid will be formed when the protein osmotic pressure is
   A. greater than the filtration pressure
   B. less than the filtration pressure
   C. the same as the filtration pressure

   a. only A
   b. A and C
   c. only B
   d. B and C

69. Major differences between extracellular and intracellular fluids are the protein content as well as sodium and potassium concentrations. Extracellular fluid contains

   a. more sodium, but less potassium and protein than intracellular fluid
   b. more sodium and potassium, but less protein than intracellular fluid
   c. less sodium and protein, but more potassium than intracellular fluid
   d. more potassium and protein, but less sodium than intracellular fluid

70. Most of the body fluid is located in the

   a. vascular compartment
   b. interstitial compartment
   c. intracellular compartment
   d. extracellular compartment

71. A number of the endocrine glands are under the control of the pituitary gland. Which of the following would fall in this group?

   A. the thyroid
   B. the ovaries
   C. the parathyroids
   D. the adrenal

   a. A and C
   b. A and B
   c. B and C
   d. C and D

72. Endocrine glands differ from salivary, sweat, and gastrointestinal glands. One major difference is that endocrine glands

   a. are ductless glands
   b. discharge their secretions through ducts
   c. are stimulated only through special sensory tracts
   d. are highly sensitive to thermal changes in the body

73. Endocrine glands secrete hormones which function in the body by

   a. initiating action of various tissues and organs
   b. regulating enzyme systems within certain tissues and organs
   c. making rapid, short term adjustments
   d. altering the heat regulatory mechanism in the body

74. All of the trophic hormones produced by the pituitary glands are of the same chemical nature. Their basic content is

   a. steroid
   b. lipid
   c. carbohydrate
   d. protein

75. The pituitary hormone which has direct effect on the reproductive system in the male is

   a. ACTH
   b. TSH
   c. FSH
   d. LTH

76. The adenohypophysis (pituitary) gland is made up of several segments of tissue. That part of the gland responsible for secreting the trophic hormones is called the

   a. pars tuberalis
   b. pars distalis
   c. pars intermedia
   d. pars nervosa

77. The secretion of antidiuretic (ADH) hormone is controlled by osmotic pressure of the blood and blood volume in the pulmonary circulation. ADH secretion increases when the

   a. osmotic pressure of blood decreases
   b. blood volume increases
   c. osmotic pressure of blood increases
   d. blood becomes diluted through large amounts of fluid ingested

78. Hormones secreted by the adrenal cortex belong to a family of chemicals called

   a. steroids
   b. glycoproteins
   c. lipids
   d. polypeptides

79. The adrenal medulla secretes two hormones, epinephrine and norepinephrine. Both of these hormones are called

   a. sympathetic agents
   b. sympathomimetic agents
   c. parasympathomimetic agents
   d. parasympathetic agents

80. Insulin is produced in the islet of Langerhans by the

    a. alpha cells
    b. beta cells
    c. gamma cells
    d. delta cells

81. The receptor organs for taste and smell are classified as

    a. pressure receptors
    b. chemical receptors
    c. thermal receptors
    d. neuro receptors

82. Although there are a number of taste sensations, only four basic qualities are recognized by the taste buds; of the four—bitter, sour, salty, and sweet—the bitter sensation is localized at the

    a. base of the tongue
    b. sides of the tongue
    c. tip of the tongue
    d. middle third of the tongue

83. The auditory tube serves the basic function of

    a. conducting sound to the outer ear
    b. equalizing air pressure within the tympanic cavity
    c. conducting sound waves from the middle to the inner ear
    d. housing the malleus, incus, and stapes

84. The decibel or one-tenth of a bel is a term customarily used for measuring the

    a. frequency of sound waves
    b. length of sound waves
    c. intensity of sound
    d. complexity of sound

85. Particles of calcium carbonate, found in the saccule and utricle, which contact sensory hair cells and record changes in the position of the head are called

    a. calcioliths
    b. otoliths
    c. equilibria stones
    d. cristae ampullaris

86. The optical system of the normal eye brings rays from distant objects into a sharp focus on the retina. On a myopic person, however, the rays focus

   a. in front of the retina
   b. behind the retina
   c. on the upper lateral border of the retina
   d. on the lower lateral border of the retina

87. As people become older they find themselves having to hold objects further away from the eyes in order to properly focus. This occurs because the

   a. lens become more elastic
   b. lens become less elastic
   c. retina becomes detached
   d. cornea becomes thickened

88. The rods and cones are specialized receptor organs of the eye. The rods are responsible for

   a. vision in high intensity light
   b. vision under conditions of low illumination
   c. general color detection
   d. vision of extremely small, delicate objects

89. Vision is the result of photochemical reactions involving the absorption of various wave lengths of light by complex light sensitive pigments. The receptor pigment of the rods is

   a. rhodopsin
   b. iodopsin
   c. photopsin
   d. scotopsin

90. The visual field for each eye is divided into two parts. The medial part (nearest the midline) is called the nasal visual field, the lateral part is called the temporal visual field. Thus, the visual cortex in the left cerebral hemisphere would receive visual impulses from objects in the

   a. temporal visual field of the left eye and the nasal visual field of the right eye
   b. temporal visual field of the right eye and the nasal visual field of the left eye
   c. temporal visual field of both the left and the right eye
   d. nasal visual field of both the left and the right eye

91. The autonomic nervous system is divided into two divisions, these are

    A. parasympathetic division
    B. sympathetic division
    C. craniosacral division
    D. thoracolumbar division
    E. sacrolumbar division

    a. A and C
    b. B and D
    c. C and D
    d. D and E

92. The shortest duration of a current necessary for excitation when its strength is twice the rheobase is called the

    a. threshold
    b. diathermy
    c. subthreshold
    d. chronaxie

93. The Hering-Breuer reflex is concerned with the regulation of

    a. respiratory inspiration
    b. pulmonary ventilation
    c. muscular contraction of the cardiac muscle
    d. taste sensation transmittal

94. The three chemicals involved in the transmission of nerve impulses are acetylcholine, epinephrine, and norepinephrine. The sympathetic transmitter agents are

    A. acetylcholine
    B. epinephrine
    C. norepinephrine

    a. A and B
    b. B and C
    c. only A
    d. A and C

95. Menopause in the older female is characterized by

    a. a decline in ovarian function
    b. a cessation in ovarian function
    c. alteration only of the external reproduction structure
    d. psychosomatic changes only

96. Carbon dioxide is carried in the blood principally in the form of

    a. bicarbonate
    b. carbonate
    c. carbohemoglobin
    d. carbamino compounds

97. Entry of food material into the respiratory tract during deglutition is prevented by

    a. elevation of the larynx
    b. elevation of the mylohyoid muscle
    c. elevation of the stomach
    d. depression of the soft palate

98. A sudden rise in carotid sinus pressure reflexly causes

    a. cardiac acceleration
    b. peripheral vasodilation
    c. peripheral vasoconstriction
    d. emptying of splenic reservoirs

99. The corpus luteum is formed

    a. immediately after ovulation
    b. only if pregnancy occurs
    c. just before ovulation
    d. at the end of the menstrual cycle

100. The basal metabolism is expressed in terms of calories per square meter of body surface per hour and is a measure of the

    a. energy required to maintain vital processes
    b. energy expended during physical exercise
    c. energy required for digestion of bland foods
    d. minimum level of cellular activity at $40°$ C

ANSWERS

1. c	11. c	21. b	31. a
2. b	12. a	22. c	32. b
3. c	13. b	23. a	33. a
4. a	14. a	24. b	34. c
5. d	15. a	25. c	35. b
6. c	16. c	26. d	36. d
7. d	17. c	27. a	37. b
8. a	18. a	28. b	38. b
9. b	19. b	29. a	39. c
10. c	20. c	30. b	40. a

41. d	56. c	71. b	86. a
42. c	57. b	72. a	87. b
43. b	58. a	73. b	88. b
44. b	59. c	74. d	89. a
45. a	60. c	75. c	90. b
46. c	61. d	76. b	91. c
47. a	62. b	77. c	92. d
48. d	63. b	78. a	93. a
49. b	64. d	79. b	94. b
50. a	65. b	80. b	95. b
51. b	66. a	81. b	96. a
52. c	67. b	82. a	97. a
53. d	68. c	83. b	98. b
54. a	69. a	84. c	99. d
55. b	70. c	85. b	100. a

REFERENCES

1. Best, C. H., and Taylor, W. B.: *The Physiological Basis of Medical Practice.* 7th Ed. Baltimore, Williams & Wilkins Co., 1961.
2. King, B. G., and Showers, M. J.: *Human Anatomy and Physiology.* 5th Ed. Philadelphia, W. B. Saunders Co., 1963.

CHAPTER 5

GENERAL ANATOMY

Henry W. Aplington, Jr. and
Katharine K. Aplington

1. Anatomy, the science of structural organization, has three main divisions: gross, microscopic, and developmental antomy. Each of these main divisions has various subdivisions, such as osteology and dermatology. The particular subdivision that is concerned primarily with the circulatory system would be known as

   a. angiology
   b. arthrology
   c. myology
   d. splanchnology

2. Another name for anatomy as studied by dissection is

   a. applied anatomy
   b. descriptive anatomy
   c. functional anatomy
   d. practical anatomy

3. The *anatomic position* is a standard, fixed position with reference to which the position of body parts is described. In this established position the

   a. body is prone
   b. hands are supinated
   c. lower limbs are abducted
   d. upper limbs are extended

4. In anatomic vocabulary, descriptive words and prefixes frequently occur in contrasting pairs, one word or prefix being the opposite of the other, for example, anterior and posterior, superficial and deep, ab- and ad-. Which of the following pairs of prefixes conforms to this scheme?

   a. a- and inter-
   b. epi- and sub-
   c. hetero- and hypo-
   d. supra- and intra-

5. If there is a structure named the *anterior superior iliac spine* (and there is, on the innominate bone), one can be reasonably certain that all of the following are also present *except* the

    a. anterior inferior iliac spine
    b. posterior inferior iliac spine
    c. posterior superior iliac spine
    d. right and left lateral iliac spines

6. A sectional plane that cuts the superior, inferior, anterior (ventral), and posterior (dorsal) aspects of the body or its parts is named a

    a. cross (or transverse) section
    b. frontal section
    c. sagittal section
    d. serial section

7. In anatomy, as in other subjects, terms should be defined as accurately as possible and employed only as defined. For example, "An organization of similar cells and their intercellular material" may be used only with reference to

    a. a region of the body
    b. an organ
    c. a tissue
    d. a system

8. The inherent segmentation of the body is quite apparent in serially homologous structures such as the vertebrae, ribs, and spinal nerves. Other structures which develop on a segmental plan, but whose segmentation later becomes masked and more difficult to see, are the

    a. hair follicles
    b. heart and lungs
    c. intestines
    d. voluntary muscles

9. An *anomaly* may be defined as a marked deviation from the normal condition occurring infrequently in occasional individuals. Some examples of anomalies are: supernumerary (extra) ribs or vertebrae, mirror image placement of organs (heart, stomach, etc.) on the opposite side of the body (this is called situs inversus), a fistula (abnormal passageway) connecting, for example, esophagus and trachea. The most satisfactory explanation and understanding of such conditions usually lies in the study of

    a. developmental anatomy
    b. microscopic anatomy
    c. physiology
    d. vestigial structures

10. Structure and function go "hand in hand." Each type of epithelial tissue, for example, is beautifully adapted to suit the functional demands of the particular surface on which it is found. Which type of epithelium forms the lining of the trachea and bronchi?

 a. pseudostratified ciliated columnar with goblet cells
 b. simple columnar striated border with goblet cells
 c. simple squamous
 d. stratified squamous, mucous type

11. Secretion, protection and temperature regulation together characterize the functional anatomy for which of the following body systems?

 a. circulatory system
 b. endocrine system
 c. integumentary system
 d. nervous system

12. A *gland* may be defined as "A cell or group of cells which regularly specializes in the formation, storage and discharge of a particular product or products." In terms of this definition, which one of the following is a gland?

 a. fibroblast cell (secretes connective tissue fibers)
 b. goblet cell (secretes mucus)
 c. simple squamous epithelial cell (secretes serous fluid)
 d. nerve cell (secretes myelin)

13. Connective tissues are variously classified into: connective tissue proper and supporting tissues, or nonskeletal and skeletal tissues, or unorganized (irregular) and organized (regular) connective tissues. An example of a supporting, skeletal, organized connective tissue would be

 a. areolar
 b. ligament
 c. tendon
 d. white fibrous

14. In contrast to epithelia, none of which are penetrated by blood vessels, all connective tissues are vascularized. Of the following connective tissues, which is the *least* vascular?

 a. areolar
 b. bone
 c. cartilage
 d. ligament

15. An aponeurosis may be defined as a broad, flat

    a. fascia
    b. ligament
    c. muscle
    d. tendon

16. Ligament and tendon connective tissue have structural features in common, but they also differ structurally in that ligament

    a. attaches to bone
    b. contains elastic fibers which allow the tissue to stretch and contract
    c. has bundles of parallel white fibers that intersect at angles
    d. is a dense type of white fibrous connective tissue

17. Generally speaking, structures that attach bones to each other are known as ligaments. Nevertheless, the term ligament is also used to designate each of the following *except* the

    a. attachment of certain abdominal organs to each other or to the abdominal wall
    b. attachment of the different parts of a muscle to each other
    c. free edge of the aponeurosis of the external oblique muscle of the abdomen
    d. remains of a fetal blood vessel such as the ductus arteriosus

18. Bone may be defined as either an organ or a tissue. Which of the following is a feature of bone considered as an organ?

    a. compact bone
    b. ground substance and white fibers
    c. periosteum
    d. spongy bone

19. Joints are classified as synarthrodial (immovable), amphiarthrodial (slightly movable), and diarthrodial (freely movable) on the basis of movability and one other feature, namely

    a. developmental type of bone present
    b. location in the body
    c. shape of the bones involved
    d. type of tissue present at the joint

20. Which of the following is a diarthrodial joint?

    a. interparietal
    b. intervertebral
    c. pubic symphysis
    d. sternoclavicular

21. Growth is increase in size, and the basis of growth is cell division. Where does the cell division occur that results in the appositional growth of a long bone?

    a. edges of the marrow cavity
    b. epiphyseal plate
    c. fibrous layer of the periosteum
    d. osteogenic layer of the periosteum

22. The formation of a primary marrow cavity is an initial phase of

    a. endochondral ossification
    b. epiphyseal ossification
    c. intramembranous ossification
    d. the repair of a bone fracture

23. Which of the following tendons properly falls within the definition of a ligament?

    a. Achilles tendon
    b. fascia lata over the quadriceps femoris muscle
    c. free aponeurotic edge of the external oblique muscle
    d. lumbodorsal aponeurosis

24. In the anatomic position, which of the bones of the superior extremity is comparable to the tibia (of the inferior extremity)?

    a. humerus
    b. radius
    c. ulna
    d. scapula

25. The dermis of the skin is composed of many structures of which some are exclusively dermal in origin while others, for example, hair follicles, are derivatives of the epidermis. Exclusively dermal structures of the skin are

    a. the arrector pili muscles
    b. the pigment granules
    c. the sebaceous glands
    d. both varieties of sweat glands

26. The superior extremity has both an extrinsic and an intrinsic musculature. An extrinsic muscle of this extremity is the

    a. coracobrachialis
    b. deltoideus
    c. supraspinatus
    d. rhomboideus

27. Generally speaking, muscles insert close to the joints they move, for example, the brachialis muscle inserts to the ulna just below the elbow joint, not distally toward the wrist. This arrangement provides

   a. greater range of movement
   b. increased leverage
   c. more power
   d. more speed

28. A given muscle may perform a variety of actions depending upon: its attachments, the independent contraction of its different parts, the action of other muscles in fixing one of its attachments so that the other attachment moves, whether or not the muscle passes over more than one joint and affects these joints differently. A muscle whose parts working together or separately may: pull the scapulae medially (retract them), or draw the scapulae upward or downward, or draw the head down on one side or directly backward is the

   a. levator scapulae
   b. rhomboideus
   c. serratus anterior
   d. trapezius

29. Which one of the following muscles passes over only one joint and produces only one action?

   a. gastrocnemius
   b. quadriceps femoris
   c. semitendinosus
   d. soleus

30. A muscle whose contraction helps to flex (forward extend) the arm is the

   a. deltoid
   b. infraspinatus
   c. latissimus dorsi
   d. triceps brachii

31. Which one of the following muscles can not possibly act as a flexor?

   a. anconeus
   b. brachioradialis
   c. brachialis
   d. supinator

32. There are four forearm muscles that insert to the wrist and produce the various motions that can occur at the wrist joint—adduction, abduction, flexion, and rotation of the hand. Which of the following pairs of muscles act as protagonists in abduction of the hand?

    a. extensor carpi ulnaris and flexor carpi radialis
    b. extensor carpi radialis and flexor carpi radialis
    c. extensor carpi ulnaris and flexor carpi ulnaris
    d. flexor carpi radialis and flexor carpi ulnaris

33. Contraction of which of the following muscles produces the action shown in Figure 2?

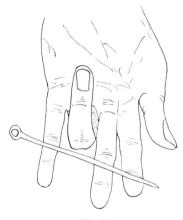

Fig. 2

    a. flexor digitorum sublimis (= superficialis)
    b. flexor digitorum profundus
    c. lumbricales
    d. ventral interosseals

34. The axilla may be defined as the region bordered laterally by the head of the humerus, medially by the serratus anterior muscle, anteriorly by the tendon of the pectoralis major, and posteriorly by the teres major muscle. Which one of the following structures changes its name when it leaves this region?

    a. axillary artery
    b. coracobrachialis muscle
    c. median nerve
    d. radial nerve

35. The term *fiber* is somewhat ambiguous because it may refer to certain cellular structures and also to certain structures that are noncellular products of cells. Which of the following are cellular structures?

    A. muscle fiber
    B. nerve fiber
    C. reticular fiber
    D. white fiber

    a. A and B
    b. B and C
    c. C and D
    d. B and D

36. Smooth muscle and skeletal muscle differ from each other in their histology, nerve supply, and general location in the body. Which of the following features are characteristic of smooth muscle?

    A. Cells are individually supplied by nerve fibers.
    B. Cells are multinucleate.
    C. Cells are lacking cross-striation.
    D. Cells receive autonomic innervation.

    a. A and B
    b. B and C
    c. C and D
    d. A and D

37. The presence of neurilemmal sheathing greatly aids the regeneration of injured nerve fibers because the neurilemmal sheath cells

    a. form a pathway along which fiber regeneration can occur
    b. form a temporary collar or splint around the injured place in the nerve
    c. nourish and protect the severed axons
    d. secrete material which helps repair of dendrites

38. Regeneration of certain nerve fibers following injury is materially aided by the presence of a neurilemmal sheath. This is particularly true of

    a. axons in peripheral nerves
    b. axons in the white matter of the central nervous system (brain and spinal cord)
    c. dendrites
    d. nonmyelinated axons

39. Approximately how many pairs of spinal nerves are present in man?

   a. 20
   b. 30
   c. 40
   d. 50

40. Which of the following structures can be dissected without cutting any bone of the vertebral column?

   a. dorsal root ganglia of spinal nerves
   b. rootlets of spinal nerves
   c. spinal nerves
   d. ventral rami of spinal nerves

41. Cell bodies of voluntary motor neurons in the spinal cord are located in the

   a. dorsal horn of the gray matter, designated by 1 in diagram
   b. lateral horn of the gray matter, designated by 2 in diagram
   c. ventral horn of the gray matter, designated by 3 in diagram
   d. white matter, designated by 4 in diagram

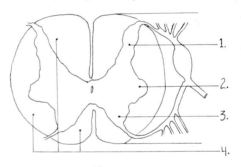

Fig. 3

42. Which contains only *motor* nerve fibers?

   a. dorsal ramus
   b. dorsal root
   c. ventral ramus
   d. ventral root

43. A *plexus* is an intermingling, or tangle, or network. To which of the following may the term *plexus* properly be applied?

   a. lymphatics
   b. nerve fibers
   c. veins
   d. all the above

44. Spinal nerves from which region of the spinal cord contribute *least* to the formation of the nerve plexuses of the limbs?

    a. cervical
    b. lumbar
    c. sacral
    d. thoracic

45. Voluntary motor nerve fibers are distributed to axial muscles of the vertebral column by way of the

    a. brachial and lumbar-sacral plexuses
    b. dorsal (posterior) root ganglia
    c. posterior rami of spinal nerves
    d. vagosympathetic trunk

46. Assume that a dorsal root of a lower cervical spinal nerve is "pinched" in some fashion, for instance by a whiplash injury, or by an arthritic spur of bone, or by a ruptured intervertebral disc. A likely symptom of this injury would be impairment

    a. in the action of one or more extensor muscles of the forearm
    b. in the action of one or more flexor muscles of the forearm
    c. in the action of the prevertebral muscles of the neck region
    d. of sensation in some area of the skin of the superior extremity

47. Definitive (emergent) nerves of the brachial plexus supply particular muscles or muscle groups of the superior extremity. Which one of the following muscle groups is supplied by the radial nerve?

    a. arm muscles that flex the forearm
    b. forearm muscles that extend the wrist and digits
    c. forearm muscles that flex the wrist and digits
    d. shoulder muscles that abduct the arm

48. What is the nerve supply of the brachialis and coracobrachialis muscles?

    a. axillary nerve
    b. median nerve
    c. middle subscapular nerve
    d. musculocutaneous nerve

49. The wall of the alimentary tube has a basic structural pattern common to its various regions: esophagus, stomach, small intestine, large intestine. In relation to special function, each of these regions also has special structural features of its own. Which of the following structures occurs in only one of these regions?

    a. goblet cells
    b. muscularis mucosae
    c. serosa
    d. villi

50. Which of these peritoneal reflections is attached to the anterior (ventral) body wall?

    a. coronary ligament of the liver
    b. falciform ligament of the liver
    c. gastro-hepato-duodenal ligament
    d. suspensory ligament of the ovary

51. What is the name of the organ (not shown here) whose position is represented by the rectangle?

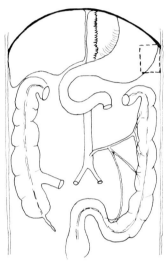

Fig. 4

    a. adrenal gland
    b. kidney
    c. pancreas
    d. spleen

52. Which one of the following structures begins and ends in capillaries?

    a. hepatic artery
    b. hepatic portal vein
    c. hepatic vein
    d. hepatic portal system

53. Functions of the liver cells are reflected by differences in concentration of substances in the hepatic portal vein as compared with the hepatic veins. Which of the following substances is usually more abundant in the hepatic veins than in the hepatic portal vein?

    a. amino acid
    b. bile salt
    c. heme
    d. urea

54. Which of the following glands have both exocrine and endocrine functions?

   A. liver
   B. pancreas
   C. testis
   D. thyroid

   a. A, B, and C
   b. B, C, and D
   c. C, D, and A
   d. D, A, and B

55. Which of these structures pass through the inguinal canal (in both males and females)?

   a. femoral artery and vein
   b. internal iliac vein
   c. peritoneum
   d. urethra

56. The right pleural cavity contains

   a. the azygous vein
   b. the lung
   c. serous fluid
   d. the thoracic aorta

57. Visualize the position of the thoracic aorta (which gives off intercostal arteries) and the azygos vein (which receives intercostal veins) in relation to the vertebral column. Which are longer?

   A. left intercostal arteries
   B. right intercostal arteries
   C. left intercostal veins
   D. right intercostal veins

   a. A and C
   b. A and D
   c. B and C
   d. B and D

58. All of the following are present in some portion or other of the mediastinal septum *except* the

   a. arch of the aorta
   b. left thoracic lymph duct
   c. thyroid gland
   d. thymus gland

59. Which of these structures is tubular, occurs in the mediastinum, and passes through the diaphragm?

    a. heart
    b. sympathetic trunk
    c. thoracic lymph duct
    d. trachea

60. The pericardial sac consists of two layers of simple squamous epithelium with some fibrous connective tissue between them. What are the names of these two layers of simple squamous epithelium?

    A. mediastinal pleura
    B. parietal pericardium
    C. parietal pleura
    D. visceral pericardium

    a. A and B
    b. B and C
    c. C and D
    d. B and D

61. The chordae tendinae are tendinous connections between the papillary muscles of the heart and the cusps of the atrioventricular valves. Which of the following best characterizes their function?

    a. to aid in preventing the return of blood to the ventricles from the aorta and pulmonary artery when these vessels contract
    b. to connect the papillary muscles with the cusps of the atrioventricular valves
    c. to ensure the closure of the bicuspid and tricuspid valves during contraction of the ventricles
    d. to open and close the atrioventricular valves

62. Assume that due to a congenital malformation of the heart some of the blood passes within the heart from one of the ventricles to the other (chiefly from left to right). This condition would be attributable to

    a. incomplete closure of the left atrioventricular valve
    b. patent ductus arteriosus
    c. patent foramen ovale
    d. patent ventricular septum

63. What is the *immediate* source of pressure that pushes blood through the coronary arteries of the heart?

    a. closure of the left atrioventricular valve
    b. closure of the semilunar valves
    c. contraction of the aorta
    d. contraction of the left ventricle

64. The heavy black in the diagram represents part of the heart's conducting system. The heart cycle begins in the sino-atrial node (upper left, in wall of opening of superior vena cava). Impulses then pass to the atrioventricular node (center, in wall of coronary sinus), and thence via the atrioventricular bundle down each side of the ventricular septum and through the moderator band of the right ventricle. Of what does this conducting system consist?

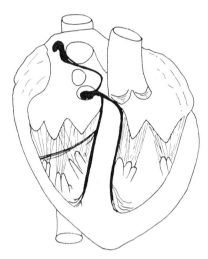

Fig. 5

a. autonomic nerve fibers
b. fibrous connective tissue specialized for conduction
c. heart muscle fibers modied to conduct impulses
d. nervous tissue intrinsic to the heart itself

65. Which one of these structural features do the largest arteries and veins have in common?

a. lumen approximately equal in diameter
b. walls consisting predominantly of elastic connective tissue
c. walls consisting predominantly of smooth muscle
d. walls having their own small blood vessels

66. Which of the following conditions is characteristic for all the veins of the body?

a. blood pressure less than atmospheric pressure
b. lined by endothelium
c. receive tributaries
d. valves are present

67. Which statement most critically characterizes a blood capillary?

    a. minute circulatory vessels through which substances can diffuse to and from the tissue fluid
    b. pertaining to or resembling a hair
    c. small blood vessels composed entirely of endothelium
    d. the many small branches of an arteriole or tributaries of a venule

68. Embolism is the sudden blocking of a blood vessel by a "floating" clot or embolus (a *thrombus* is a clot remaining at its place of formation). If an embolus originated in the left spermatic or ovarian vein and stopped in the first capillaries it came to, in which of these organs would it lodge?

    a. brain
    b. heart
    c. kidney
    d. lung

69. The fluid part of the blood, that is, the noncellular part of the blood, is named

    a. lymph
    b. plasma
    c. serum
    d. tissue fluid

70. Veins lack pulse because

    a. a capillary bed intervenes between arteries and veins
    b. other factors aid the flow of blood in veins
    c. their walls are flabby and distensible
    d. pulse ends in the arterioles

71. Which of the following is a polymorphonuclear cell that has cytoplasmic granules, is ameboid, and is produced in the bone marrow?

    a. erythrocyte
    b. monocyte
    c. neutrophilic leukocyte
    d. thrombocyte

72. Which of the following terms is defined as a temporary increase in the number of circulating white blood cells?

    a. anemia
    b. leukemia
    c. leukocytosis
    d. polycythemia

73. Which of the following regularly participates in the transport of carbon dioxide in the blood?

    a. erythrocytes
    b. leukocytes
    c. thrombocytes
    d. none of the above

74. Most of the diffusion of tissue fluid from the intercellular spaces into circulatory vessels takes place via the

    a. arterial capillaries
    b. lymph capillaries
    c. venous capillaries
    d. thin walls of venules

75. Which of the following regularly occurs more abundantly per unit volume in tissue fluid and less abundantly per unit volume in lymph?

    a. amino acids
    b. fibrinogen
    c. lymphocytes
    d. saturated fats

76. Lymph nodes occur in the course of lymph vessels and consist of lymphatic tissue. What does lymphatic tissue consist of?

    A. lymph
    B. lymphocytes
    C. reticular connective tissue
    D. tissue fluid

    a. A and B
    b. B and C
    c. C and D
    d. A and C

77. Fluid which enters the kidney tubules (via Bowman's capsule) is

    a. lymph
    b. plasma
    c. tissue fluid
    d. urine

78. Urea is manufactured by cells of the

    a. kidney
    b. large intestine (colon)
    c. liver
    d. skin

79. It is a principle that involuntary effectors (smooth muscle, cardiac muscle, and glands) of the body receive two sets of autonomic nerve fibers (parasympathetic and sympathetic). Which one of the following structures receives only sympathetic innervation and is therefore an exception to this general rule?

    a. blood vessels
    b. ciliary muscle of the eye
    c. kidney
    d. lung

80. The behavior of involuntary effectors is a compromise between the opposing effects of parasympathetic and sympathetic stimulation. Which of the following is a result of predominantly parasympathetic stimulation?

    a. dilation of the bronchioles
    b. pupil of the eye becomes smaller
    c. reduced salivary gland secretion
    d. speed of blood clotting is increased

81. Which one of the following organs contains striated muscle that is involuntary (supplied by autonomic nerve fibers)?

    a. aorta
    b. esophagus
    c. lung
    d. stomach

82. Cell bodies of preganglionic sympathetic neurons are located in the

    a. brain
    b. dissectible ganglia along or connected with the sympathetic trunk
    c. lateral horn of gray matter of the thoracic and lumbar spinal cord
    d. ventral horn of the gray matter of the spinal cord

83. *All* of the following muscles assist in protraction of the mandible. All of them also assist in elevation of the mandible *except* the

    a. external pterygoid
    b. internal pterygoid
    c. masseter
    d. temporal

84. The name of the indicated muscle is the

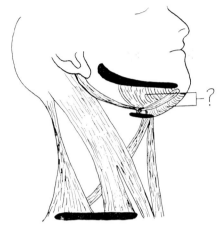

Fig. 6

   a. geniohyoid
   b. mylohyoid
   c. omohyoid
   d. sternohyoid

85. To which one of the following categories of head muscles does the digastric muscle of man belong?

   a. facial
   b. jaw
   c. throat
   d. tongue

86. Which of the following pharyngeal derivatives develops from the epithelial floor of the pharynx (rather than from one or more of the pharyngeal pouches or arches)?

   a. parathyroid gland
   b. thymus gland
   c. thyroid gland
   d. tonsil

87. Which of these skull foramina transmits three of the twelve cranial nerves and is located between the temporal and sphenoid bones?

   a. foramen ovale
   b. internal auditory meatus
   c. jugular foramen
   d. stylomastoid foramen

88. Dural sinuses are large, anastomosing, noncollapsible channels between the layers of the dura mater of the brain. These channels contain

    a. blood with a high oxygen content
    b. blood with a low oxygen content
    c. cerebrospinal fluid
    d. lymph

89. The heavy line indicates the lateral or sylvian fissure of the cerebrum This fissure forms a separation between the

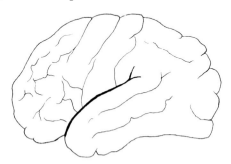

Fig. 7

    a. parietal and occipital lobes
    b. precentral and postcentral gyri
    c. temporal and frontal lobes
    d. two cerebral hemispheres

90. Which part of the brain produces neurosecretions that pass to the pituitary gland and stimulate its hormonal activity?

    a. cerebral hemispheres
    b. hypothalamus
    c. medulla oblongata
    d. superior colliculi

91. Centers for the regulation of appetite and thirst are contained in the

    a. cerebrum
    b. medulla
    c. midbrain
    d. hypothalamus

92. The cerebral aqueduct or aqueduct of Sylvius is a tubular communication between the

    a. fourth ventricle and the subarachnoid space
    b. lateral ventricles and the third ventricle
    c. third ventricle and the fourth ventricle
    d. two lateral ventricles

93. Unlike spinal nerves, all of which contain both sensory and motor nerve fibers, only some of the cranial nerves have a mixed fiber content. Other cranial nerves are either sensory only or motor only. Which of the following is a mixed cranial nerve?

    a. facial VII
    b. hypoglossal XII
    c. optic II
    d. trochlear IV

94. All of the following cranial nerves contain sensory fibers that begin in taste buds and transmit taste sensation *except* the

    a. facial VII
    b. glossopharyngeal IX
    c. trigeminal V
    d. vagus X

95. The following structures are all modifications or reflections of the dura mater *except* the

    a. corpus callosum
    b. falx cerebri
    c. sclerotic coat and cornea of the eye
    d. tentorium cerebelli

96. The posterior lobe of the pituitary body is composed of

    a. pars anterior and pars tuberalis
    b. pars intermedia and pars anterior
    c. pars neuralis and pars anterior
    d. pars neuralis and pars intermedia

97. Which of the following structures forms a separation between the anterior and posterior chambers of the eye?

    a. lens
    b. iris
    c. ciliary muscle
    d. visual layer of the retina

98. The "sound sensitive" hair cells of the inner ear are located in the

    a. ampullae of the semicircular canals
    b. organ of Corti
    c. utriculus and sacculus
    d. scala vestibuli

99. The nasal passageways are to the perpendicular plate of the ethmoid what the lateral ventricles are to the

    a. massa intermedia
    b. septum pellucidum
    c. falx cerebri
    d. optic chiasma

100. A frontal section (of the head) that passes through the frontal lobe of the brain, the posterior part of the eyeball, the nasal passageways, and the hard palate would also pass through the

    a. maxillary sinus
    b. parotid gland
    c. oropharynx
    d. pituitary gland

101. Which of the following structures would be cut by a midsagittal section of the head?

    a. cerebral peduncle
    b. internal ear
    c. occipital condyle
    d. tuber cinereum

ANSWERS

1. a	21. c	41. c	61. c
2. d	22. a	42. d	62. d
3. b	23. c	43. d	63. c
4. b	24. c	44. d	64. c
5. d	25. a	45. c	65. d
6. c	26. d	46. d	66. b
7. c	27. d	47. b	67. c
8. d	28. d	48. d	68. d
9. a	29. d	49. d	69. b
10. a	30. a	50. b	70. d
11. c	31. a	51. d	71. c
12. b	32. b	52. d	72. c
13. b	33. a	53. d	73. a
14. c	34. a	54. a	74. c
15. d	35. a	55. c	75. a
16. c	36. c	56. c	76. b
17. b	37. a	57. c	77. c
18. c	38. a	58. c	78. c
19. d	39. b	59. c	79. a
20. d	40. d	60. a	80. b

81. b	86. c	91. d	96. d
82. c	87. c	92. c	97. b
83. a	88. b	93. a	98. b
84. b	89. c	94. c	99. b
85. c	90. b	95. a	100. a
			101. d

REFERENCES

1. Anson, B. J.: *Morris' Human Anatomy*. 12th Ed. New York, McGraw-Hill, 1966.
2. Aplington, H. W., Jr.: *Principles of Anatomy—A Text and Laboratory Guide*. Columbus, The Hollenback Press, 1966.
3. Crouch, J. E.: *Functional Human Anatomy*. Philadelphia, Lea & Febiger, 1965.
4. Edwards, L. F.: *Concise Anatomy*. 2nd Ed. New York, McGraw-Hill, 1956.
5. Ham, A. W.: *Histology*. 5th Ed. Philadelphia, J. B. Lippincott, 1965.

CHAPTER 6

CHEMISTRY

C. Keith Claycomb

1. Elements that have the same atomic number but different atomic weights are called

    a. isobars
    b. isotopes
    c. radioactive
    d. protons

2. Metallic oxides react with water to form

    a. bases
    b. amines
    c. neutral salts
    d. acids

3. Which of the following are physical properties of substances?

    A. noncombustible
    B. color
    C. reactivity toward substances
    D. density
    E. solubility in various solvents

    a. only D
    b. A and C
    c. A, D, and C
    d. B, D, and E

4. Which of the following are chemical properties of a substance?

    A. noncombustible
    B. color
    C. reactivity toward substances
    D. density
    E. solubility in various solvents

    a. only A
    b. A and C
    c. A, D, and C
    d. B, D, and E

5. Examples demonstrating the transformation of energy are

    A. burning of wood
    B. generation of electrical power
    C. winding of a clock
    D. rubbing your hands together

    a. A and C
    b. B and D
    c. A, B, and D
    d. all are correct

6. The simplest compounds are those formed by the union of

    a. two molecules
    b. an isotope and isobar
    c. two elements
    d. sodium and nitric acid

7. The process by which a fire is self-ignited is called

    a. enthalpy
    b. entropy
    c. kindling temperature
    d. spontaneous combustion

8. A process which always occurs along with oxidation is

    a. smoke production
    b. reduction
    c. light production
    d. heat liberation

9. A way in which temporary hard water may be softened is by

    a. acidifying
    b. neutralizing
    c. freezing
    d. boiling

10. Mixtures in which individual molecules of the solute are uniformly dispersed throughout the solvent are known as

    a. true solutions
    b. colloidal solutions
    c. suspensions
    d. emulsions

11. Mixtures of solute and solvents in which the former will settle out upon standing are known as

    a. true solutions
    b. colloidal solutions
    c. suspensions
    d. emulsions

12. Approximately how many kilograms are there in a pound?

    a. 0.45
    b. 1.05
    c. 4.50
    d. 10.00

13. The process by which a substance in solution distributes itself uniformly throughout the solvent is called

    a. depression
    b. diffusion
    c. osmosis
    d. suspension

14. An acid is best defined as any substance that is a donor of

    a. hydrogen ions
    b. hydronium ions
    c. hydroxide ions
    d. protons

15. When a chemist refers to an acid as strong or weak, he is referring to its

    a. concentration
    b. degree of ionization
    c. halogen ion content
    d. oxygen content

16. To convert centigrade temperature to Fahrenheit, it is necessary to

    a. multiply by 5/9 and add 32
    b. multiply by 5/9 and subtract 32
    c. multiply by 9/5 and subtract 32
    d. multiply by 9/5 and add 32

17. Approximately how many kilocalories would be liberated if a gallon of water at 100°F. were cooled to freezing (0°C.)?

    a. 10
    b. 41.7
    c. 100
    d. 143

18. Air is a mechanical mixture of many gaseous substances. Which one of the components given is *not* utilized by some animal or bacteria?

    a. CO_2
    b. O_2
    c. N_2
    d. none of the above, i.e., all are used

19. An atom of the lightest element would contain the following particles

    A. electron
    B. proton
    C. neutron

    a. only A
    b. only B
    c. A and B
    d. B and C

20. An atom which contained a total of ten electrons would be

    a. an inert gas
    b. a metal
    c. a molecule
    d. a radioisotope

21. What is the combining valence of nitrogen in the compound $NaNO_3$?

    a. -6
    b. $+5$
    c. -4
    d. $+3$

22. Which one of the following is a correctly balanced equation for a possible reaction?

    a. $Ca + Cl_2 \rightarrow CaCl_2$
    b. $K + O \rightarrow KO_2$
    c. $S + 2Fe \rightarrow Fe_2S$
    d. $H_2 + Cl \rightarrow H_2Cl$

23. Which of the following elements exist as molecules in the free state under standard conditions?

    A. chlorine
    B. fluorine
    C. helium
    D. neon
    E. oxygen

    a. A and D
    b. B and C
    c. A, B, and E
    d. all are correct

24. Which type(s) of chemical valence(s) is (are) present in ammonium chloride?

    A. coordinate covalence
    B. covalence
    C. electrovalence

    a. only C
    b. A and B
    c. B and C
    d. all are correct

25. When potassium chlorate is heated, oxygen is liberated and potassium chloride is formed. Which of the following is a correct and balanced equation for this reaction?

    a. $2KClO_3$ (+heat) $\rightarrow$ $2KCl + 3O_2$
    b. KCl_2O_2 (+heat) $\rightarrow$ $KCl_2 + O_2$
    c. K_2ClO (+heat) $\rightarrow$ $K_2Cl + O$
    d. $KClO_3$ (+heat) $+ KCl + O_2$

26. What gas is liberated when sodium carbonate reacts with sulfuric acid?

    a. CO
    b. CO_2
    c. SO_2
    d. SO_3

27. Conditions which favor reactions going to completion are the formation of

    A. an electrolyte
    B. a gas
    C. an insoluble product
    D. water

    a. A and D
    b. B and C
    c. B, C, and D
    d. all are correct

28. Oxidation may be defined as a

    A. gain of electrons
    B. loss of electrons
    C. loss of hydrogen
    D. gain of oxygen
    E. loss of oxygen

    a. A and D
    b. B and E
    c. A, C, and E
    d. B, C, and D

29. Which of the following substances contribute to hardness of water?

    A. ions of heavy metals
    B. ions of light metals
    C. carbonates
    D. chlorides

    a. only B
    b. A and C
    c. B and D
    d. A, C, and D

30. The selective flow of a solvent through a semi-permeable membrane (one that the solute cannot pass through) is called

    a. diffusion
    b. dispersion
    c. osmosis
    d. suspension

31. Colloidal particles are large enough to display surface phenomena, and as such they

    a. carry an electrical charge
    b. are electrically neutral
    c. are the same size as solutes of true solution
    d. settle out upon standing

32. What is (are) common to all halogens?

    A. They all react with water to form bases.
    B. They all react with water to form acids.
    C. They all react with metals to form salts.
    D. They all have seven electrons in their outer valence shell.

    a. B only
    b. A and C
    c. C and D
    d. B and D

33. How many gram-molecular weights of sulfur would be needed to react completely with a gram-molecular weight of iron to form ferrous sulfide?

    a. 0.5
    b. 1.0
    c. 1.5
    d. 3.0

34. What is the approximate normality of an aqueous solution prepared by dissolving 10 grams of NaOH in a total volume of 100 ml.?

    a. 0.15
    b. 2.5
    c. 6.0
    d. 8.2

35. What is the approximate normality of a solution prepared by diluting 500 ml. of 5.0 N HCl to one liter with distilled water?

    a. 0.15
    b. 2.5
    c. 6.0
    d. 8.2

36. What is the approximate normality of concentrated hydrochloric acid whose specific gravity is approximately 1.2 and is 38% HCl by weight?

    a. 2.5
    b. 6.0
    c. 8.2
    d. 12.4

37. Approximately how many grams of NaOH would be required to neutralize 12 ml. of the acid (HCl) in problem No. 36?

    a. 2.5
    b. 6.0
    c. 8.2
    d. 12.4

38. Clinical studies have shown that in temperate zones, 1 ppm of fluoride added to drinking water is effective in reducing dental decay in children. Which of the following represents approximately 1 ppm of fluoride in water?

    A. 1.0 mg. of F^- per liter
    B. 2.2 mg. of NaF per liter
    C. 2.08 mg. of NaF per quart
    D. 1 oz. of NaF in 3.4 gallons

    a. only A
    b. A and C
    c. B, C, and D
    d. all are correct

39. Which of the following salts, when dissolved in distilled, neutral water, would have a hydrogen (hydronium) ion concentration greater than 1×10^{-7} gram-moles per liter?

    A. sodium acetate
    B. sodium bicarbonate
    C. sodium chloride
    D. monobasic sodium phosphate
    E. ammonium chloride

    a. only B
    b. A and C
    c. D and E
    d. A, B, and C

40. Approximately how many times more hydrogen (hydronium) ions are present in a liter of 0.001 HCl than a liter of a solution of pH 3?

    a. 2
    b. 3
    c. 4
    d. 0

41. One element that all organic compounds contain is

    a. carbon
    b. nitrogen
    c. oxygen
    d. sulfur

42. Compounds that have the same molecular formulas but differ in their properties are called

    a. carbohydrates
    b. hydrocarbons
    c. isomers
    d. isotopes

43. Compounds which contain only carbon and hydrogen are called

    a. carbohydrates
    b. hydrocarbons
    c. optical isomers
    d. proteins

44. Which of the given names would be correct for the pictured organic compound?

$$CH_3C(CH_3)CH_3$$
$$|$$
$$Cl$$

   A. 2-chloro-2-methyl propane
   B. trimethyl chloromethane
   C. tertiary butyl chloride

   a. only A
   b. only C
   c. A and B
   d. all are correct

45. Both ethanol and phenol contain a hydroxy radical. Yet only phenol will react with NaOH because

   a. ethanol is a weak base
   b. phenol is a weak base
   c. ethanol is a weak acid
   d. phenol is a weak acid

46. Which one of the following compounds could exhibit optical activity?

   a. $HOOC-CH_2-COOH$
   b. $CH_3-CO-COOH$
   c. $CH_3-CH(OH)-COOH$
   d. $H_2C = CH-COOH$

47. How many different compounds have the following formula?
$$C_5H_{12}$$

   a. 1
   b. 2
   c. 3
   d. 4

48. Which one of the halogen derivatives of the methane series is an easily liquified gas and is used as a safe refrigerant?

   a. CH_3Cl
   b. $CHCl_3$
   c. $C_2H_4Br_2$
   d. CCl_2F_2

49. Ethene has a greater reactivity toward halogens than does ethane because

    a. ethane reactions are of the addition type
    b. ethane reactions are of the substitution type
    c. ethene is easily oxidized to ethane
    d. ethene is an unsaturated compound

50. An illuminating gas may be produced by the addition of water to

    a. CaC_2
    b. $CaCO_3$
    c. $(CH_3COO)_2Ca$
    d. calcium oxalate

51. Compounds whose formula is C_nH_n (where n is a finite number) are always

    A. aromatic compounds
    B. cyclic compounds
    C. hydrocarbons
    D. unsaturated compounds

    a. only C
    b. A and D
    c. C and D
    d. all are correct

52. What are common properties of compounds with the formula $R-CH_2-O-CH_2-R'$?

    A. all are gases at room temperature (25°C)
    B. almost all may be used as anesthetics
    C. all are highly inflammable
    D. all readily form salts with sodium

    a. only A
    b. B and C
    c. A and D
    d. all are correct

53. Oxidation of a compound with the formula of C_3H_8O formed acetone. Therefore, the original compound must have been

    a. methyl-ethyl ether
    b. ethoxy ethane
    c. isopropyl alcohol
    d. n-butyl alcohol

54. Which of the following are true about alcohols?

    A. They all contain at least one OH group.
    B. They are all very reactive.
    C. They are all liquids at room temperature.
    D. They are all produced by fermentation.

    a. only A
    b. only C
    c. B and D
    d. all are correct

55. All soaps

    A. are metallic salts of fatty acids
    B. form true (aqueous) solutions
    C. are good emulsifying agents

    a. only A
    b. only C
    c. B and C
    d. all are correct

56. Soaps that form opalescent colloidal mixtures in water and are good emulsifying agents are

    A. hard soaps
    B. insoluble soaps
    C. soft soaps
    D. soluble soaps

    a. only D
    b. A and B
    c. C and D
    d. A, C, and D

57. The polymerization of chloroprene (2-chloro-1, 3-butadiene) under controlled conditions results in the formation of

    a. butadiene
    b. GR-N
    c. GR-S
    d. neoprene

58. The position that a new group will occupy when added to a benzene ring is influenced by the group already present. Therefore, if bromo-benzene were nitrated, where would the $-NO_2$ group be located with respect to the bromine?

    A. ortho
    B. meta
    C. para

    a. only B
    b. only C
    c. A and B
    d. A and C

59. If nitrobenzene were to be brominated, where would the Br be located in respect to the $-NO_2$ group? (Refer to general discussion in No. 58.)

    A. ortho
    B. meta
    C. para

    a. only B
    b. only C
    c. A and B
    d. A and C

60. Partial reduction of acetone would give

    a. n-propyl alcohol
    b. 2-propanol
    c. lactic acid
    d. acetic acid

61. A 10% solution of formalin is used to preserve tissues for histologic studies. To prepare one liter of 10% formalin one would use

    a. 330 ml. 30% aqueous formic acid solution and dilute to one liter
    b. 150 ml. of formalin and dilute to one liter
    c. 250 ml. of 40% aqueous solution of formaldehyde and dilute to one liter
    d. 100 gm. of acetaldehyde and dilute to one liter

62. Vinegar is a

    A. dilute solution of acetic acid
    B. weak acid
    C. dilute solution of vinyl acetate

    a. only A
    b. only C
    c. A and B
    d. B and C

63. In general, the physical properties of fatty acids are due to their carbon chain length. Therefore, as the length increases the acids

    A. become less water soluble
    B. become more greasy
    C. exhibit a higher melting point
    D. become more soluble in organic solvents

    a. only A
    b. only B
    c. C and D
    d. all are correct

64. When one talks about polyunsaturated cooking oils, he is actually referring to

    a. the degree of hydrogen saturation of the fatty acid components
    b. how much unsaturated glycerol is present
    c. a tristearate
    d. those that contain a large amount of fatty acids of 6 carbon atoms or less

65. The valence of nitrogen in the quaternary ammonium germicides is

    a. 1
    b. 3
    c. 5
    d. 7

66. The empirical formula of benzene (C_6H_6) indicates that it is an unsaturated hydrocarbon. However, it does not act like one in that benzene is very stable and most reactions are substitutions rather than addition types. A paramount reason for this stability is the existence of

    a. double bonds
    b. normal bond lengths between carbon atoms
    c. resonance
    d. unsaturation

67. The compounds formed by the saponification of a fat are

    A. soaps
    B. glycerol
    C. fatty acids
    D. sodium glycerate

    a. A and B
    b. A and D
    c. B and C
    d. all are correct

68. One thing that nitroglycerin and T.N.T. have in common is that both

    A. are explosives
    B. contain three nitro groups per molecule
    C. contain glycerol
    D. are hydrocarbons

    a. only A
    b. A and B
    c. A, C, and D
    d. all are correct

69. The only amino acid that does not contain an asymmetric carbon atom and therefore cannot be designated as either 'L' or 'D' configuration is

    a. arginine
    b. glycine
    c. lysine
    d. proline

70. It is difficult to produce a lather using sodium palmitate in permanently hard water possibly because

    a. sodium palmitate is not a soap
    b. the dissolved halogens interfere with the organic compound
    c. the dissolved heavy metals form insoluble palmitate compounds
    d. sodium palmitate is a low sudsing detergent

71. The food substance which constitutes the mainstay of civilized man's diet is

    a. carbohydrate
    b. fat
    c. lipid
    d. protein

72. What cation is essential for normal blood coagulation?

    a. Ca^{+2}
    b. Cl^{-1}
    c. CN^{-1}
    d. Fe^{+2}

73. Nucleic acids are required for protein synthesis. Which one transfers genetic information from the nucleus to the cytoplasmic ribosomes?

    a. messenger DNA
    b. transfer DNA
    c. messenger RNA
    d. transfer RNA

74. The process of combining CO_2 and H_2O, utilizing the energy of the sun and chlorophyll of plants to give carbohydrates and O_2, is

    a. glucolysis
    b. gluconeogenesis
    c. phototropism
    d. photosynthesis

75. The treatment of disease by chemical substances is known as

    a. biochemistry
    b. chemotherapy
    c. cybernetics
    d. cryotherapy

76. A specific aldohexose is

    a. arabinose
    b. fructose
    c. glucose
    d. maltose

77. A disaccharide which is also a reducing sugar is

    a. fructose
    b. glucose
    c. maltose
    d. sucrose

78. A sugar which consists of equal amounts of glucose and fructose is

    a. arabinose
    b. lactose
    c. maltose
    d. sucrose

79. Glucose is stored by animals as the polysaccharide

    a. cellulose
    b. dextrin
    c. glycogen
    d. starch

80. A pathway by which the body can catabolize glucose without finally using the tricarboxylic acid cycle (T.C.A.) is the

    a. carbon cycle
    b. hexose monophosphate shunt
    c. Krebs-Henseleit urea cycle
    d. pyruvic acid cycle

81. Complete hydrolysis of starch, dextrin, glycogen, and cellulose all yield one compound which is

    a. fructose
    b. glucose
    c. glycerol
    d. a ketohexose

82. Compounds that are classified as lipids are

    A. cephalins
    B. fats
    C. fatty acids
    D. lecithins

    a. only B
    b. only C
    c. B and C
    d. all are correct

83. The main building blocks of proteins are organic acids which have a specific group substituted on their alpha carbon. With the exception of two acids, this group is always a (an)

    a. ammonium ion
    b. primary amine
    c. secondary amine
    d. tertiary amine

84. The currency of the body, that is the energy necessary for doing work, is due to high energy phosphate bonds. Which of the following contain high energy bonds?

A. ADP
B. ATP
C. creatine phosphate
D. glucose-1-phosphate

a. only B
b. B and D
c. A, B, and C
d. all are correct

85. The final oxidation of fats, carbohydrates, and proteins is primarily accomplished by one common pathway. This metabolic course is the

a. carbon cycle
b. Krebs-Henseleit urea cycle
c. pyruvic acid cycle
d. tricarboxylic acid cycle

86. The first step in the catabolism of fat is its hydrolysis into glycerol and fatty acids. The glycerol may then be metabolized by carbohydrate pathways. Complete oxidation of the fatty acids is by

a. beta oxidation and the tricarboxylic acid cycle
b. beta oxidation
c. the tricarboxylic acid cycle
d. anaerobic glycolysis

87. Substances which are produced by ductless glands and carried by the blood to another organ where they influence its metabolism are known as

a. essential amino acids
b. hormones
c. metabolites
d. substrates

88. A nitrogen-containing acid which occurs only in connective tissue and predominantly in collagen is

a. hydroxyproline
b. lysine
c. phenylalanine
d. tryptophan

89. An analysis of the gastric contents of a sick patient showed the presence of fermented carbohydrates and native (undigested) proteins. Therefore, the problem could be due to

A. deficiency of parietal cell secretion
B. deficiency of chief cell secretion
C. excessive amounts of ptyalin secretion
D. excessive amounts of carbohydrate ingestion

a. only A
b. A and B
c. C and D
d. B, C, and D

90. What is the approximate biologic caloric value of 75 gm. of a food that is composed of 75% water, 8% protein, 4% fat, and 13% carbohydrate? (Answers are given in large calories.)

a. 7 Cal.
b. 70 Cal.
c. 90 Cal.
d. 120 Cal.

91. The oxidation of the primary alcohol group of glucose would give

a. glucaldaric acid
b. gluconic acid
c. glucosaccharic acid
d. glucuronic acid

92. The advantage that an animal incurs by storing carbohydrates as a polysaccharide instead of as glucose is

A. less water is needed (reduced osmotic effect)
B. the animal can convert fat into glycogen more easily than into glucose
C. less ATP is required per mole of glucose for glycolysis than for glucolysis
D. it is easier to absorb the glycogen from the blood stream

a. only A
b. only B
c. A and C
d. B and D

93. Pellagra, a deficiency disease, occurs in those whose main food source is some form of corn. A plausible explanation for this is

    A. deficiency of a B vitamin
    B. the corn protein, zein, is deficient in certain essential amino acids
    C. corn is deficient in niacin

    a. only A
    b. only B
    c. only C
    d. all are correct

94. An enzyme is a protein, or a protein and a nonprotein (co-enzyme) complex. Which of the following (is) are correct statement(s) about enzymes?

    A. their specificity is due to the protein
    B. many of the co-enzymes have a vitamin as an integral part
    C. a co-enzyme may be involved in more than one reaction depending upon its associated protein
    D. substances which denature (modify) proteins could interfere with enzymatic reactions

    a. only A
    b. only B
    c. A, C, and D
    d. all are correct

95. We have the following set of reactions occurring in the body, and each step (A, B, C and D) is catalyzed by an enzyme. If enzyme C is blocked by a chemical inhibitor, one would expect that the following would occur.

$$f$$
$$A \quad B \Updownarrow \quad C \quad D$$
$$a \rightleftharpoons b \rightleftharpoons c \rightleftharpoons d \rightleftharpoons e$$
$$\Updownarrow$$
$$g$$

    A. The concentration of d would remain the same.
    B. The concentration of substance c would rise.
    C. The concentration of substance b would rise.
    D. The concentration of substance b would be unaffected.
    E. Death to the organism could result.

    a. only A
    b. A and C
    c. B and E
    d. A, C, and D

96. Serum albumin has an isoelectric point of 4.88. Which of the following is (are) true about this protein in blood (pH = 7.4)?

    A. It would have maximum solubility if the blood pH were dropped to pH of 4.88.

    B. It would have a net positive charge.

    C. It is an anion.

    a. only A
    b. only B
    c. only C
    d. A and B

97. A sample of human blood failed to coagulate within a normal time period. Which of the following is (are) a plausible reason(s) for this noncoagulation?

    A. The sample vial had been treated with dicoumarin before the blood sample was added.

    B. The sample vial had been treated with silicone before the blood sample was added.

    C. The blood donor had been on dicoumarin therapy.

    D. The blood donor had been on vitamin K therapy.

    a. only A
    b. only B
    c. A and D
    d. B and C

98. If one mole of an ideal gas at standard conditions occupies 22.4 liters, what volume would two moles of this same gas occupy at 2 atmospheres and 0°C.?

    a. 1 x 22.4 liters
    b. 2 x 22.4 liters
    c. 3 x 22.4 liters
    d. 4 x 22.4 liters

99. The overall reaction

$$_{92}^{235}U + _0^1n \rightarrow \, _{92}^{236}U \rightarrow \, _{63}^{150}Eu + _{35}^{80}Br + 4\,_0^1n + 6\,beta$$
particles

is an example of

    A. nuclear fission
    B. nuclear fusion
    C. transmutation
    D. radioactive emission

    a. only A
    b. only B
    c. A, C, and D
    d. B, C, and D

100. When 2.50 grams of hydrated barium chloride were heated, the resulting anhydrous powder weighed 2.13 gm. Therefore, you know that the

    A. formula for the hydrated salt is $BaCl_2 \cdot 7H_2O$
    B. percentage of water in the hydrated salt is 14.8
    C. hydrated salt was a dihydrate
    D. number of moles of anhydrous $BaCl_2$ produced is 1.03×10^{-2}

    a. only A
    b. A and D
    c. A, B, and D
    d. B, C, and D

ANSWERS

1. b	26. b	51. c	76. c
2. a	27. c	52. b	77. c
3. d	28. d	53. c	78. d
4. b	29. b	54. a	79. c
5. d	30. c	55. a	80. b
6. c	31. a	56. c	81. b
7. d	32. c	57. d	82. d
8. b	33. b	58. d	83. b
9. d	34. b	59. a	84. c
10. a	35. b	60. b	85. d
11. c	36. d	61. c	86. a
12. a	37. b	62. c	87. b
13. b	38. d	63. d	88. a
14. d	39. c	64. a	89. a
15. b	40. d	65. c	90. c
16. d	41. a	66. c	91. d
17. d	42. c	67. a	92. c
18. d	43. b	68. b	93. d
19. c	44. d	69. b	94. d
20. a	45. d	70. c	95. c
21. b	46. c	71. a	96. c
22. a	47. c	72. a	97. d
23. c	48. d	73. c	98. a
24. d	49. d	74. d	99. c
25. a	50. a	75. b	100. d

REFERENCES

1. Arnow, L., and Logan, M.: *Introduction to Physiological and Pathological Chemistry*. 6th Ed. St. Louis, C. V. Mosby Co., 1961.
2. Bogert, L. J.: *Fundamentals of Chemistry*. 9th Ed. Philadelphia, W. B. Saunders Co., 1963.

CHAPTER 7

PHARMACOLOGY

Nancy J. Reynolds

1. Pharmacology is defined as
   a. the study of actions, both beneficial and harmful, of all substances upon the body
   b. the science which treats of the origin, the nature, and the effects of drugs
   c. the study of drugs used in the treatment of the sick
   d. the study of drugs used in the diagnosis of disease

2. Official drugs are those listed in the
   A. United States Pharmacopeia, which is published by the American Pharmaceutical Association
   B. United States Pharmacopeia, which is revised every five years
   C. National Formulary, which is revised every ten years
   D. National Formulary, which is published by the American Pharmaceutical Association

   a. A and D
   b. B and D
   c. A and C
   d. B and C

3. The Pharmacopeia of the United States and the National Formulary were designated as the official standards for drugs by
   A. an act of Congress
   B. the Federal Food, Drug, and Cosmetic Act
   C. the Department of Health, Education, and Welfare
   D. the National Bureau of Standards

   a. A and B
   b. A and C
   c. A and D
   d. only A

4. The dispensing and possession of narcotics are regulated by

    A. the Department of Internal Revenue
    B. restriction to licensed physicians, dentists, and veterinarians
    C. the Harrison Narcotic Act which has never been amended
    D. the American Medical Association

    a. A and B
    b. B and C
    c. C and D
    d. all of the above

5. There are several ways by which a drug may be designated as to name. These include which of the following?

    A. the generic name, which is the chemical formula
    B. the generic name, which reflects the chemical name and is never changed
    C. the official name, which is the only one listed in the *Accepted Dental Remedies*
    D. the brand name, which is assigned by the manufacturer

    a. A and D
    b. B and D
    c. A and C
    d. B and C

6. A drug is defined as

    a. a synthetic substance used in the diagnosis, treatment, or prevention of disease
    b. any chemical substance which produces an action and effect on body tissues
    c. anything which cures, palliates, or prevents disease
    d. a refined material used in therapeutics

7. Pharmacologically active compounds found in plants are grouped according to their physical and chemical properties. Examples of these are

    a. alkaloids, which have a bitter taste
    b. oils (fixed only)
    c. parenteral
    d. topical

8. The characteristic of volatile oils that distinguishes them from fixed oils is

    A. they are greasy to the touch
    B. they are soluble in alcohol
    C. they evaporate readily
    D. they are readily soluble in water

    a. A and B
    b. A and C
    c. C and D
    d. B and C

9. Emulsions and mixtures differ in that

    a. only emulsions are suspensions
    b. mixtures contain an agent for dispersing the droplets of oil
    c. only mixtures have an aqueous vehicle
    d. mixtures are suspensions of insoluble nonfatty solids in water; emulsions contain fats or oil suspended in water

10. The difference between (1) liniments and lotions, and (2) emollients and demulcents is that

    a. group one is used exclusively on skin
    b. group one contains no active ingredient
    c. only group two promotes healing
    d. only group two contains oil

11. A liter of 2 ppm solution contains what quantity of the drug?

    A. 2 mg.
    B. 20 mg.
    C. .002 Gm.
    D. .02 Gm.

    a. A and C
    b. B and C
    c. A and D
    d. B and D

12. Which of the following reflect the more pertinent factors in determining the dosage of a drug?

    A. the age rather than the metabolism
    B. the size rather than the sex
    C. the metabolism rather than the size
    D. the sex rather than the age

    a. A and B
    b. B and C
    c. A and D
    d. all of the above

13. What must be added to the following statement to make it correct? Metabolism is measured by the amount of O_2 the patient utilizes per unit of body surface, per given time

    a. at normal activity
    b. per body weight
    c. under sedation
    d. at rest

14. The greatest hazard to the patient in the administration of drugs by injection is

    a. an improperly sterilized needle
    b. breakage of a needle
    c. failure to aspirate
    d. failure to cleanse the tissue prior to injection

15. Which of the following abbreviations used in prescription writing indicate the time of day a drug should be administered?

    A. h.s.
    B. p.c.
    C. q.s.
    D. q.

    a. A and C
    b. B and C
    c. A and B
    d. all of these

16. In prescription writing, which of the following parts are specifically required *only* when the drug ordered is a narcotic?

    A. subscription
    B. location of doctor's office
    C. license number of the doctor
    D. registered number of the doctor

    a. A and D
    b. A and C
    c. B and C
    d. B and D

17. One of the oldest of the barbiturates is Luminal. Which of the following statements pertains to this drug?

    a. It is a long-acting drug known also as pentobarbital sodium.
    b. It is widely used as preoperative medication for elderly patients.
    c. It is a short-acting drug, is used as a general anesthetic agent, and is rarely given orally.
    d. It is known also as phenobarbital sodium, acts over a long period of time, and acts specifically on the motor cortex of the brain.

18. Sodium pentothal and methohexital sodium differ fundamentally in that

    a. one is a sedative, the other a vasodilator
    b. one acts over a longer period of time
    c. one is given intramuscularly, the other intravenously
    d. one makes an alkaline solution, the other acidic, when mixed with water

19. Which of the following drugs can be used for the control or treatment of convulsive attacks?

    A. bromides
    B. phenobarbital
    C. Dilantin sodium
    D. Mesantoin

    a. A, B, and C
    b. A, C, and D
    c. A, B, C, and D
    d. only C and D

20. A substance administered orally or parenterally, which contains no pharmacological agent and to which any response is purely psychic, is called

    a. a cerate
    b. a placebo
    c. a tranquilizer
    d. an emollient

21. A patient has been given repeated therapeutic doses of pentobarbital sodium and atropine sulfate. The patient is a highly nervous individual with liver disease and a history of diabetes. After eighteen hours, the patient manifests the symptoms of a barbiturate overdose. The response is most likely to be a result of

    a. synergism
    b. potentiation
    c. cumulation
    d. hypersensitivity

22. The therapeutic actions of opium are due to which components?

    A. Laudanum
    B. morphine
    C. salts
    D. alkaloids

    a. A and D
    b. A and C
    c. B and C
    d. B and D

23. Methylmorphine is the narcotic of choice for the treatment of

    a. coronary occlusion
    b. emphysema
    c. a gastric ulcer
    d. a cough

24. The dosage of methylmorphine is

    a. 30 mg.
    b. gr. 1/6
    c. 100 mg.
    d. 3 mg.

25. Analgesia and sedation differ in that

    a. only sedatives act on the cerebrum
    b. analgesia means absence of pain, and sedation means loss of consciousness
    c. analgesia means absence of sensitivity to pain, and sedation means a reduced response to irritating stimulation
    d. only analgesics depress respiration

26. A derivative of morphine which is non-narcotic and which is a vasodilator is

    a. physostigmine
    b. papaverine
    c. paraldehyde
    d. phenothiazine

27. A derivative of morphine which competes with narcotics for the cell receptors, thereby antagonizing the action of the initial drug is

    a. nalorphine
    b. neostigmine
    c. nikethamide
    d. Dilaudid

28. A fluid extract differs from a tincture in that

    a. a fluid extract is an alcoholic preparation, but a tincture is an aqueous one
    b. the final volume of a fluid extract is adjusted so that each cc. contains 1 gm. of drug, whereas a tincture is adjusted so that each cc. contains 0.5 gm. of drug
    c. a fluid extract is a derivative of a plant drug, whereas a tincture is always a derivative of a synthetic substance
    d. the final volume of a fluid extract is adjusted so that each cc. contains 1 gm. of drug, whereas a tincture is adjusted so that each cc. contains 0.1 or 0.2 gm. of drug

29. In converting dosages from grains to milligrams, it is necessary to

    a. divide by 15

    b. multiply by 15

    c. divide by 60

    d. multiply by 60

30. The difference between cubic centimeters and milliliters is

    A. very slight

    B. significant

    C. of no practical significance

    D. approximately one ounce

    a. A and D

    b. A and C

    c. B and C

    d. B and D

31. To make a 100% solution, add

    a. 1 gm. of the drug to enough solvent to make 1 cc. of solution

    b. 10 gm. of the drug to 10 cc. of solvent

    c. 50 gm. of the drug to enough solute to make 5 cc. of solution

    d. 1 gm. of the drug to 1 cc. of solvent

32. Meperidine hydrochloride is a synthetic analgesic and is the drug of choice over morphine in a dental office because

    A. it is a more effective pain reliever

    B. it diminishes salivary flow in addition to its analgesic effect

    C. it does not cause addiction

    D. it produces less respiratory depression

    a. A and C

    b. A and D

    c. B and C

    d. B and D

33. Which of the following are non-narcotic synthetic analgesics?

    A. propoxyphene hydrochloride

    B. phenacetin

    C. acetylsalicyclic acid

    D. meperidine hydrochloride

    a. A, B, and C

    b. A, C, and D

    c. B, C, and D

    d. all of these

34. Dosage of acetylsalicylic acid is
    A. 10 gr. q. 4 h.
    B. 5 gr. q. 2 h.
    C. 600 mg. q. 4 h.
    D. 300 mg. q. 2 h.

    a. A and B
    b. B and D
    c. A and C
    d. all of these

35. Antipyretics reduce an elevated body temperature by
    a. action on the heat regulation center in the spinal cord
    b. increasing the elimination of heat
    c. constriction of peripheral blood vessels
    d. acting on the carotid body

36. The toxic or allergic reactions to aspirin include
    a. urticaria which is subcutaneous extravasation
    b. angioneurotic edema which is swelling without inflammation or infection
    c. leukopenia which is an increase in white blood cells
    d. anti-inflammatory response

37. The salicylates are used as anti-inflammatory agents in treating
    a. chronic infections
    b. periodontosis
    c. rheumatic fever
    d. typhoid fever

38. Amphetamine, which is prepared synthetically from ephedrine, is a central nervous system stimulant and therefore useful as
    A. an agent to combat fatigue
    B. a restorative agent in respiratory depression
    C. a drug to treat hypertension
    D. an ataractic

    a. A and D
    b. B and D
    c. A and C
    d. A and B

39. Dextroamphetamine is a derivative of amphetamine and is frequently prescribed to
    a. decrease the rate of metabolism
    b. counteract hypertension
    c. depress the appetite
    d. depress salivary secretions

40. The nervous system that regulates the heart, smooth muscle, and glands is called

    a. the sympathetic nervous system
    b. the autonomic nervous system
    c. the central nervous system
    d. the brain stem

41. The postganglionic fibers of the parasympathetic nervous system release, at their terminals, a substance which facilitates the transmission of impulses. This chemical is known as

    a. adrenalin
    b. sympathin
    c. epinephrine
    d. acetylcholine

42. The ganglia of the sympathetic nervous system are located

    a. on or near the organ they innervate
    b. close to the central nervous system
    c. in the spinal cord
    d. in the brain stem

43. Which of the nervous systems largely controls involuntary functions concerned with mass response to unusual stimuli?

    a. autonomic
    b. peripheral
    c. parasympathetic
    d. sympathetic

44. What type of drug is epinephrine?

    A. adrenergic
    B. sympathomimetic
    C. a hormone
    D. an enzyme

    a. A and B
    b. A, B, and D
    c. only A
    d. A, B, and C

45. The actions of epinephrine include

    A. moderate vasoconstriction
    B. increased heart rate
    C. relaxation of smooth muscle of the respiratory tract
    D. constriction of bronchiole musculature

    a. A and D
    b. A and C
    c. B and C
    d. B and D

46. Epinephrine is used in dentistry to
    a. control massive hemorrhage
    b. intensify and prolong the action of the local anesthetic agents
    c. facilitate absorption of local anesthetic agents
    d. provide all of the above

47. Which of the following drugs are similar in action to, but appreciably safer than, epinephrine, and which can be given orally?
    A. Neo-Synephrine
    B. Levophed
    C. ephedrine
    D. Neo-Cobefrin

    a. A, B, and C
    b. B, C, and D
    c. A, C, and D
    d. A, B, and D

48. The cholinergic blocking agents which belong to the belladonna group of drugs include
    A. pilocarpine
    B. atropine
    C. neostigmine
    D. scopolamine

    a. A and B
    b. A and C
    c. B and C
    d. B and D

49. The actions of atropine sulfate include
    A. acceleration of heart rate
    B. decreased secretions
    C. resultant amnesia
    D. increased salivation

    a. A and B
    b. A and C
    c. A and D
    d. A, B, and D

50. Drugs which block the ganglia of the sympathetic nervous system have what effect on the parasympathetic ganglia?
    a. no effect
    b. same effect
    c. opposite effect
    d. exaggerated effect

51. Neostigmine and physostigmine produce what effect upon the body?

    a. cholinergic
    b. adrenergic
    c. anticholinergic
    d. sympathomimetic

52. Histamine is similar to epinephrine in that it

    a. is a powerful dilator of capillaries
    b. occurs naturally in the body
    c. causes a rise in blood pressure
    d. regulates pulse rate

53. An antigen is a substance which stimulates the human organism to produce

    a. antihistamine
    b. hormones
    c. antibodies
    d. enzymes

54. Acquired hypersensitivity means that the individual will exhibit

    a. an over-response to a drug
    b. an allergic response to the induction of a particular antigen
    c. certain psychic manifestations in response to drug administration
    d. a sensitivity reaction to penicillin

55. Anaphylactic reaction is

    a. the allergic response to a substance in which rash, sneezing, and angioneurotic edema are produced
    b. the violent attack of symptoms in a hypersensitive patient which could result in death
    c. any allergic response
    d. the development of blood dyscrasias following administration of a drug

56. Which of the following are useful antihistamines with their correct dosage?

    A. Pyribenzamine hydrochloride 250 mg. q. 4 h.
    B. diphenhydramine hydrochloride 25 to 50 mg.
    C. Phenergan hydrochloride 25 mg.
    D. Benadryl hydrochloride 25 to 50 mg.

    a. A and B
    b. A, B, and C
    c. B, C, and D
    d. only D

57. Certain antihistaminic drugs are also useful to prevent or control the symptoms of

   A. inner ear dysfunctions
   B. motion sickness
   C. radiation sickness
   D. diarrhea

   a. A, B, and C
   b. A, B, and D
   c. A, C, and D
   d. B, C, and D

58. Motion sickness is the result of inability to tolerate

   a. continuous horizontal movements
   b. intermittent horizontal movements
   c. continuous vertical movements
   d. intermittent vertical movements

59. Caffeine is used to combat fatigue and occasionally as a respiratory stimulant since it acts as

   a. a central nervous system depressant
   b. an analgesic
   c. a stimulant of the cerebrum and medullary centers
   d. an innervator of the cerebellum

60. Nikethamide is an analeptic which is particularly useful in combating respiratory depression. It is also known as

   a. Coramine
   b. Metrazol
   c. Ritalin
   d. Megimide

61. Picrotoxin as an analeptic must be used with caution because it is

   A. highly toxic
   B. a sedative
   C. a convulsant
   D. a central nervous system depressant

   a. A and B
   b. A and C
   c. B and D
   d. B and C

62. The fatal dosage of caffeine is 10 gm. If a cup of coffee contains 200 mg. of caffeine, this means the fatal dose would be approximately how many cups? (one teacup contains 6 fluid ounces).

    a. 50
    b. 5
    c. 500
    d. 550

63. Antibacterial agents of chemical origin which are used systemically are called chemotherapeutic agents. Similar agents of biologic origin are called

    a. antitoxins
    b. antiseptics
    c. antibiotics
    d. anticoagulants

64. Penicillin is not effective against

    A. gram-positive bacteria
    B. some gram-negative organisms
    C. true viruses
    D. streptococci

    a. A and D
    b. B and C
    c. A and C
    d. B and D

65. Toxic reactions to penicillin include

    A. chills
    B. diarrhea
    C. dermatitis
    D. joint pains

    a. A, C, and D
    b. B, C, and D
    c. A, B, and D
    d. all of the above

66. Allergic reactions to penicillin include

    a. convulsions
    b. muscular twitching
    c. joint pains
    d. asthma

67. One of the greatest problems in penicillin therapy is

    a. the toxic reactions
    b. the appearance of resistant strains of bacteria
    c. its instability in solution
    d. its selective action

68. To increase its effectiveness, oral penicillin may be given

    A. in large doses
    B. with a buffering agent
    C. several times a day
    D. at mealtime

    a. A, B, and C
    b. A, C, and D
    c. B, C, and D
    d. all of the above

69. Which of the following are tetracycline compounds and are listed with the correct generic name?

    a. Aureomycin (oxytetracycline)
    b. Achromycin (tetracycline)
    c. neomycin (erythromycin)
    d. Erythrocin (erythromycin)

70. The dosage of most of the "mycin" drugs is usually

    A. 250 mg. q.i.d.
    B. 1 gm. b.i.d.
    C. 250 mg. q.6 h.
    D. 1 gm. per day in divided doses

    a. A, B, and C
    b. A, B, and D
    c. A, C, and D
    d. B, C, and D

71. Broad-spectrum antibiotics are indicated

    a. in any infection other than viral
    b. in most gram-negative bacilli infections
    c. for patients sensitive to the tetracyclines
    d. for the treatment of thrush

72. Chloramphenicol (Chloromycetin) is the antibiotic which is most effective against

    a. tuberculosis
    b. dysentery
    c. typhoid fever
    d. cholera

73. In the treatment of tuberculosis the drug of choice is

   a. streptomycin
   b. neomycin
   c. chloramphenicol
   d. bacitracin

74. The most serious toxic reaction to chloramphenicol is

   a. anaphylaxis
   b. agranulocytosis
   c. deafness
   d. superinfection

75. The most serious toxic response to streptomycin is

   a. anaphylaxis
   b. deafness
   c. diarrhea
   d. phlebitis

76. Erythromycin is most similar to which one of the following drugs in its range of antibacterial activity?

   a. Aureomycin
   b. neomycin
   c. penicillin
   d. Achromycin

77. The sulfa drugs act by competing with the vitamin B component which is essential for bacterial metabolism. This component is

   A. para-aminobenzoic acid
   B. the parent compound of Novocain
   C. para-aminosalicyclic acid
   D. meta-aminobenzoic acid

   a. A and D
   b. A and B
   c. A and C
   d. only C

78. The properties of certain sulfa drugs render them safer and more effective than others. These properties include

   A. relative insolubility in body fluids
   B. rapid absorption from the intestine
   C. solubility in urine
   D. rapid excretion

   a. A and C
   b. A and B
   c. B and D
   d. B and C

79. The advantage of the triple sulfa mixtures is that

    a. a larger amount of each drug can be administered safely
    b. the danger of renal blockage is reduced
    c. elimination through the liver is facilitated
    d. the solubility of each drug is enhanced

80. The Rauwolfia compounds are the drugs of choice for a patient who exhibits

    a. emotional disturbances with resulting hypertension
    b. low blood pressure
    c. emotional disturbances with resulting hypotension
    d. high blood pressure

81. Phenergan (promethazine hydrochloride) has what pharmacologic properties?

    A. antihistaminic
    B. ataractic
    C. emetic
    D. potentiation of analgesics

    a. A, B, and D
    b. A, C, and D
    c. B, C, and D
    d. all of the above

82. Which of the following are ataractics?

    A. meprobamate
    B. chloramphenicol
    C. Compazine
    D. diphenhydramine

    a. A, B, and C
    b. A, C, and D
    c. A and D
    d. A and C

83. Which of the following preparations produce(s) hemostasis?

    A. thrombin
    B. oxidized cellulose
    C. heparin
    D. epinephrine

    a. A, B, and C
    b. A, B, and D
    c. A, B, C, and D
    d. only A

84. Vitamin K affects coagulation by

   a. producing fibrin
   b. acting in the synthesis of prothrombin
   c. precipitating blood proteins
   d. constriction of capillaries

85. Astringents are useful in checking capillary bleeding because they

   a. coagulate blood proteins
   b. provide a network for fibrin
   c. constrict the severed ends of arterioles
   d. are mechanical protectives

86. Eugenol is obtained from which essential oil?

   a. oil of peppermint
   b. oil of clove
   c. oil of wintergreen
   d. oil of orange

87. Zinc oxide and eugenol, as a protective dressing, acts as

   a. an obtundent
   b. a counterirritant
   c. a desiccating agent
   d. a sterilizing agent

88. Hydrogen peroxide solution as a mouthwash should be used with great caution because it

   a. kills certain anaerobic microorganisms
   b. tends to produce granulation tissue
   c. has a pH of 3
   d. has a pH of 10

89. Amyl nitrite is used to relieve anginal pain because it is

   a. an analgesic
   b. a sedative
   c. a vasodilator
   d. a vasoconstrictor

90. Aromatic spirits of ammonia acts as

   a. a reflex respiratory stimulant
   b. a reflex cardiac depressant
   c. a vasodilator
   d. an antispasmodic

91. Cortisone is an anti-stress drug and is a hormone produced

    a. only synthetically
    b. in the adrenal gland
    c. in the cerebral cortex
    d. in the anterior pituitary gland

92. Which of the following are local anesthetic agents derived from para-aminobenzoates?

    A. procaine (Novocain)
    B. tetracaine (Pontocaine)
    C. metabutoxycaine (Primacaine)
    D. lidocaine (Xylocaine)

    a. A and D
    b. A and C
    c. A and B
    d. B and D

93. The most dangerous complication in administering local anesthetic agents is usually a result of

    a. correct technique but toxic response to the agent
    b. breakage of the needle
    c. septic equipment
    d. accidental intravenous injection

94. Lidocaine hydrochloride differs from Novocain in which of the following properties?

    a. Potency is not as great.
    b. Duration of anesthesia is longer.
    c. More concentrated solutions are essential.
    d. Toxicity is considerably less.

95. Mepivacaine is marketed as

    a. Unacaine
    b. Carbocaine
    c. Monocaine
    d. butethamine

96. Mepivacaine is available in a 2% solution containing

    a. epinephrine 1:100,000
    b. epinephrine 1:50,000
    c. Neo-Cobefrin 1:20,000
    d. Neo-Cobefrin 1:50,000

97. Which one of the following agents is under the regulation of the Harrison Narcotics Law?

    a. Nupercaine
    b. cocaine
    c. Metycaine
    d. ethyl chloride

98. If a local anesthetic of short duration is required, the drug of choice would be

    a. lidocaine
    b. Carbocaine
    c. Monocaine
    d. Unacaine

99. The chief disadvantage of Pontocaine hydrochloride is its

    a. relative impotency
    b. increased toxicity
    c. long duration
    d. low affinity for nerve tissue

100. Propoxycaine hydrochloride (Ravocaine) is used in conjunction with procaine in order to provide

    a. anesthesia of short duration
    b. fewer toxic responses
    c. rapid, more profound anesthesia of long duration
    d. slower onset of symptoms

101. Vasopressors added to local anesthetic agents provide which of the following advantages?

    A. prolonged duration of anesthesia
    B. dilated vessels thereby increasing rapid dispersion of drugs
    C. reduced quantity of agent needed
    D. elimination of the need to aspirate

    a. A and D
    b. A and C
    c. A and B
    d. all of the above

102. Topical anesthetics are effective for

    a. producing local surface analgesia prior to injection
    b. limited surgery in deep tissues of the oral cavity
    c. producing counterirritation to ulcerated areas
    d. reducing toxicity of other agents

103. If a patient is allergic to Novocain, which surface anesthetic would be indicated.

    a. benzocaine
    b. lidocaine ointment
    c. pontocaine solution
    d. butacaine

104. Agents used in the administration of general anesthesia in the dental office include

    A. barbiturates
    B. inhalation agents
    C. muscle relaxants
    D. anticholinergic drugs

    a. A and B
    b. A, B, and C
    c. A, B, C, and D
    d. only A

105. Requirements of an ideal intravenous agent for producing unconsciousness include

    A. slow induction
    B. provision of adequate duration of effect for completion of the procedure
    C. slow recovery without nausea
    D. complete reversibility of effects

    a. A and B
    b. B and C
    c. B and D
    d. only B

106. Thiopental sodium, which is frequently referred to as Pentothal sodium, exhibits which of the following properties?

    A. destroyed rapidly (chiefly by the liver)
    B. has some analgesic effect
    C. produces laryngospasms in many patients
    D. lowers blood pressure in therapeutic doses

    a. A and D
    b. B and C
    c. C and D
    d. A and C

107. What is the most important aspect of any general anesthetic?

    a. Anesthesia must be profound enough for the completion of the procedure.

    b. No hypoxia must occur.

    c. The patient must recover rapidly.

    d. No painful stimuli must be introduced until the correct level of anesthesia is reached.

108. Muscle relaxants are used in conjunction with general anesthesia in order to achieve

    a. an adequate level of anesthesia in a light plane

    b. inhibition of respirations, thereby decreasing requirements of large volumes of inhalation agents

    c. analgesia

    d. greater laryngeal responses

109. Which of the following muscle relaxants exhibit the same mechanism of action?

    A. curare

    B. Syncurine

    C. Anectine

    D. Quelicin

    a. B, C, and D

    b. A and D

    c. A, B, and C

    d. all of the above

110. The most important requirement for administering general anesthesia in a dental office is

    a. adequate equipment

    b. properly trained personnel

    c. emergency equipment

    d. a great variety of drugs

111. The most frequent and most dangerous complication in general anesthesia is

    a. sudden circulatory collapse

    b. an overdose of anesthetic agent

    c. an obstructed airway

    d. prolonged apnea

112. Which of the following inhalation agents is (are) nonexplosive, has (have) a great margin of safety for the dental office, is (are) inorganic compound(s) (contains no carbon atoms), and has (have) low anesthetic potency?

    A. ethylene
    B. cyclopropane
    C. nitrous monoxide
    D. N$_2$O

    a. A and B
    b. B and C
    c. C and D
    d. only B

113. Divinyl ether has what advantage over diethyl ether?

    a. wider margin of safety
    b. more rapid in onset of anesthesia
    c. less toxic
    d. less expensive

114. Which inhalation agent used to supplement nitrous oxide forms a poisonous gas when in contact with soda-lime?

    a. Vinethene
    b. cyclopropane
    c. Trilene
    d. fluothane

ANSWERS

1. b	17. d	33. a	49. a
2. b	18. b	34. d	50. b
3. a	19. c	35. b	51. a
4. a	20. b	36. b	52. b
5. b	21. c	37. c	53. c
6. b	22. d	38. d	54. b
7. a	23. d	39. c	55. b
8. d	24. a	40. b	56. c
9. d	25. c	41. d	57. a
10. a	26. b	42. b	58. c
11. a	27. a	43. d	59. c
12. b	28. d	44. d	60. a
13. d	29. d	45. c	61. b
14. c	30. b	46. b	62. a
15. c	31. a	47. c	63. c
16. d	32. d	48. d	64. b

65. c	78. d	91. b	104. c
66. d	79. b	92. c	105. c
67. b	80. a	93. d	106. d
68. a	81. a	94. b	107. b
69. b	82. d	95. b	108. a
70. c	83. b	96. c	109. a
71. b	84. b	97. b	110. b
72. c	85. a	98. d	111. c
73. a	86. b	99. b	112. c
74. b	87. a	100. c	113. b
75. b	88. c	101. b	114. c
76. c	89. c	102. a	
77. b	90. a	103. b	

REFERENCES

1. Accepted Dental Remedies. 30th Ed. Council on Dental Therapeutics, American Dental Association, 1965.
2. Adriani, J.: *The Chemistry of Anesthesia.* Springfield, Charles C Thomas, 1959.
3. Dobbs, E. C.: *Pharmacology and Oral Therapeutics.* 12th Ed. St. Louis, C. V. Mosby Co., 1961.
4. Dobbs, E. C., and Prinz, H.: *Pharmacology and Dental Therapeutics.* 10th Ed. St. Louis, C. V. Mosby Co., 1951.
5. Falconer, M. W., and Norman, M. R.: *The Drug, The Nurse and the Patient.* Philadelphia, W. B. Saunders Co., 1958.
6. Krug, E. E.: *Pharmacology in Nursing,* 9th Ed. St. Louis, C. V. Mosby Co., 1963.
7. Kutscher, A. H., Zegarelli, E. V., Hyman, G. A., McLean, P., and Kutscher, H. W.: *Pharmacology for the Dental Hygienist.* Philadelphia, Lea & Febiger, 1967.
8. Mack, E., Garrett, A. B., Haskins, J. F., and Verhoek, F. H.: *Textbook of Chemistry.* 2nd Ed. Boston, Ginn and Co., 1958.
9. Winton, F. R., and Bayliss, L. E.: *Human Physiology.* 5th Ed. New York, McGraw-Hill, 1962.
10. Wright, H. N., and Montag, M. L.: *A Textbook of Pharmacology and Therapeutics.* 7th Ed. Philadelphia, W. B. Saunders Co., 1959.

CHAPTER 8

NUTRITION

Babette Graf

1. Complete proteins are supplied by
    a. cottage cheese, cereal, milk, and beef
    b. cottage cheese, egg, milk, and beef
    c. jello, cottage cheese, milk, and cereal
    d. olive, cheese, cereal, and milk

2. Which one of the following substances is an essential amino acid?
    a. pyruvic acid
    b. linoleic acid
    c. glycine
    d. methionine

3. Which one of the following classifications applies to the protein of gelatin?
    a. complete protein
    b. partially complete protein
    c. incomplete protein
    d. conjugated protein

4. Of the following foods, which one is a pure protein food?
    a. egg yolk
    b. egg white
    c. lean beef
    d. milk

5. Which one of the substances listed below contains the reference protein?
    a. milk
    b. beef
    c. egg
    d. fish

6. The requirement for protein is influenced by

   A. an individual's activity
   B. an individual's environment
   C. an individual's age
   D. an individual's total carbohydrate intake

   a. A and D
   b. B and C
   c. C and D
   d. all of the above

7. Kwashiorkor, the most widespread protein deficiency, affects mainly

   2.
   a. children just weaned
   b. children 6 to 12 years old
   c. teenagers
   d. pregnant women

8. What part of the total energy intake in the United States is supplied by protein in the diet?

   a. 14 to 16%
   b. 20 to 25%
   c. 30 to 40%
   d. 40 to 50%

9. Which one of the Basic Four Food Groups is almost devoid of protein?

   a. dairy products
   b. meats
   c. vegetables and fruits
   d. breads and cereals

10. Mutual supplementation of dietary protein is represented by which one of the following examples?

   a. corn and navy-beans
   b. beef and navy-beans
   c. milk and navy-beans
   d. egg and navy-beans

11. If taken by mouth, which one of the following carbohydrates can furnish energy almost immediately?

   3.
   a. sucrose
   b. lactose
   c. glucose
   d. fructose

12. The carbohydrate occurring naturally in milk is called

    a. glucose
    b. fructose
    c. maltose
    d. lactose

13. Good sources of cellulose are obtainable from which of the following foods?

    a. white bread, potatoes, carrots, and crackers
    b. carrots, lettuce, cake, and honey
    c. carrots, rice, prunes, and cornflakes
    d. bran, spinach, cabbage, and green beans

14. Carbohydrates are stored for future needs as

    a. glycerol
    b. glycogen
    c. fatty acids
    d. amylase

15. The average carbohydrate content in the diet of the average person in the United States is

    a. 10% of the total calories
    b. 30% of the total calories
    c. 50% of the total calories
    d. 70% of the total calories

16. The end products of carbohydrate metabolism are

    a. carbon dioxide and urea
    b. carbon dioxide and water
    c. carbon dioxide, water, and urea
    d. carbon dioxide and ammonia

17. Of the following foods, which group contains the highest starch content?

    a. milk, egg, potato, and rice
    b. bread, tomato, rice, and table sugar
    c. cornmeal, navy-beans, rice, and potato
    d. cornmeal, banana, olive, and green beans

18. The part of the cereal grain which contains the highest percentage of nutrients is located in the

    a. bran
    b. germ
    c. endosperm
    d. husk

19. Of the following foods, which ones are broken down to glucose only in the digestive tract?

    a. rice, salad oil, egg white and honey
    b. rice, cornstarch, cake flour and tapioca
    c. rice, pineapple juice, chocolate candy and egg whites
    d. orange, tomato juice, cake flour and rice

20. A teaspoon of sucrose weighing 10 gm. furnishes the body with

    a. 5 Calories
    b. 10 Calories
    c. 20 Calories
    d. 40 Calories

21. According to the Basic Four Food groups, the recommended daily intake of bread is

    a. 3 slices
    b. 4 slices
    c. 5 slices
    d. 6 slices

22. Which of the following foods yield *only* fatty acids and glycerol during digestion?

    A. eggs
    B. lard
    C. olive oil
    D. honey

    a. A and B
    b. B and C
    c. C and D
    d. all of the above

23. Linoleic acid belongs to the group of substances known as

    a. amino acids
    b. fatty acids
    c. bile acids
    d. sterols

24. The substance essential for the absorption of fats is

    a. lipoprotein
    b. bile
    c. lipase
    d. maltase

25. When glucose is not metabolized for energy, the substance that will accumulate in the blood stream is

    a. amino acids
    b. bile acids
    c. keto acids
    d. phytic acid

26. Of the following foods, the one that has the highest fat content is

    a. corn oil
    b. peanut butter
    c. cheese (American)
    d. pork chop

27. The nutritional difference between white whole milk and skim dry milk is the

    a. energy, vitamin A, and riboflavin content
    b. energy and vitamin A content
    c. energy, vitamin A, and ascorbic acid content
    d. energy, vitamin A, and fat content

28. If the curtailing of fats in a diet is desired, the following group of foods should be eliminated

    a. rice, milk, jello, and olives
    b. rice, olives, apple pie, and eggs
    c. mayonnaise, salmon, bacon, and peanut butter
    d. french fried potatoes, milk, syrup, and herring

29. The phospholipid found in egg yolk is called

    a. cephalin
    b. stearin
    c. lecithin
    d. casein

30. Of the different body fats, the greatest percentage comprises the group known as

    a. cholesterol
    b. neutral fats
    c. phospholipids
    d. waxes

31. Five grams of butter contain

    a. 20 Calories
    b. 25 Calories
    c. 45 Calories
    d. 50 Calories

32. Factors that affect basal metabolism are

    A. growth

    B. mental activity

    C. surface area

    D. sex

    a. A, B, and D

    b. A, B, and C

    c. A, C, and D

    d. all of the above

33. Glycerol and fatty acids result from the digestive breakdown of

    a. egg white

    b. orange

    c. butter

    d. potato

34. The nature of insulin is that of

    a. a hormone

    b. an enzyme

    c. a vitamin

    d. a mineral

35. The hormone that influences energy metabolism is called

    a. pepsin

    b. thyroxine

    c. lactase

    d. cortisone

36. The enzyme amylase breaks down

    a. starch

    b. sucrose

    c. protein

    d. neutral fats

37. Carbohydrate digestion takes place mainly in

    a. the mouth and the stomach

    b. the mouth

    c. the stomach

    d. the small intestine

38. Dipeptides are related to

    a. proteins

    b. fats

    c. carbohydrates

    d. minerals

39. The enzyme trypsin is necessary for the digestion of

    a. carbohydrates
    b. fats
    c. proteins
    d. vitamin B_{12}

40. Protein digestion is started in which one of the following organs?

    a. mouth
    b. stomach
    c. duodenum
    d. small intestine

41. The first enzyme that acts on mayonnaise which has just been ingested is

    a. amylase
    b. pepsin
    c. trypsin
    d. lipase

42. Two-thirds of the National Research Council's recommended allowance of calcium for adults is furnished by consuming

    a. one cup of white whole milk
    b. two cups of white whole milk
    c. three cups of white whole milk
    d. four cups of white whole milk

43. An outstanding source of calcium is

    a. bread
    b. butter
    c. egg
    d. American cheese

44. Of the following substances, those that are poorly absorbed are

    A. amino acids
    B. calcium
    C. glucose
    D. iron

    a. A and B
    b. B and C
    c. B and D
    d. A and D

45. Spinach contains which of the following nutrients?

    A. calcium, methionine, lecithin
    B. iron, folic acid, maltose
    C. folic acid, calcium, ascorbic acid
    D. vitamin A, folic acid, iron

    a. A and B
    b. B and C
    c. C and D
    d. all of the above

46. The Recommended Dietary Allowances for iron have been set at

    a. double the amount needed by the body
    b. five times the amount needed by the body
    c. three times the amount needed by the body
    d. ten times the amount needed by the body

47. The mineral necessary for the prevention of goiter is

    a. thyroxine
    b. iodine
    c. iron
    d. fluorine

48. To safeguard dental health, the amount of fluorine added to water must be at least

    a. 1 ppm
    b. 1 ml./l.
    c. 1 c./gal.
    d. 1 mg./lb.

49. Which two of the following substances are functionally related?

    a. phosphorus and calcium
    b. fluorine and iron
    c. calcium and iron
    d. sodium and phosphorus

50. The nutritional deficiencies which contribute to rickets are

    a. calcium and vitamin A
    b. calcium and vitamin D
    c. fluorine and vitamin A
    d. fluorine and vitamin D

51. The foods in which the best sources of vitamin A are found would be

    a. carrots, tomato, milk, and spinach
    b. tomato, bread, corn, and beef
    c. wheatflour, cucumber, red beets, and peas
    d. tea, squash, apples, and tomato

52. The preferred storage depot for vitamin A in the human body is

    a. plasma
    b. bone
    c. liver
    d. skin

53. Of the following substances, the precursor of vitamin A in the body is

    a. ergosterol
    b. cholesterol
    c. carotene
    d. glucose

54. If a physician would be prescribing a supplementary vitamin pill containing vitamin A for a small child, the proper dosage (R.D.A. = 2000) would be

    a. 1,800 I.U.
    b. 5,000 I.U.
    c. 10,000 I.U.
    d. 12,500 I.U.

55. The vitamin which is part of the enzyme co-carboxylase is called

    a. niacin
    b. riboflavin
    c. thiamine
    d. pantothenic acid

56. Of the following foods, which is the best source of thiamine?

    a. pork
    b. orange
    c. potato
    d. white milk

57. Beriberi is a condition caused by a deficiency of the vitamin called

    a. niacin
    b. riboflavin
    c. thiamine
    d. pantothenic acid

58. Under the enrichment act, a substance which must be added to white flour is

    a. vitamin A
    b. vitamin D
    c. ascorbic acid
    d. thiamine

59. The part of riboflavin supplied by one cup of white milk for an adult woman's Recommended Dietary Allowance is

    a. ¼ the recommended daily allowance
    b. ⅓ the recommended daily allowance
    c. ½ the recommended daily allowance
    d. ⅔ the recommended daily allowance

60. Of the following foods, which one is the best source of riboflavin?

    a. beef liver
    b. cabbage
    c. whole wheat bread
    d. tomato

61. The enzyme FAD, containing riboflavin, functions in the area of

    a. hydrogen transport
    b. protein digestion
    c. blood clotting
    d. B_{12} absorption

62. The food which furnishes the greatest amount of niacin equivalents is

    a. enriched bread
    b. spinach
    c. milk
    d. egg

63. The amino acid, which is converted to niacin by the human body, is

    a. valine
    b. methionine
    c. tryptophan
    d. lysine

64. Milk is almost entirely lacking in

    a. thiamine
    b. ascorbic acid
    c. riboflavin
    d. tocopherol

65. Vitamin C is not essential for the function of

    A. wound healing
    B. tooth formation
    C. energy metabolism
    D. carbohydrate digestion

    a. A and B
    b. B and C
    c. C and D
    d. all of the above

66. The cheapest source of ascorbic acid in household portions is obtained from

    a. canned tomato juice
    b. milk
    c. strawberries
    d. green peppers

67. A person suffering from night blindness should be advised to consume a large quantity of

    a. eggs, cauliflower, potatoes, and apples
    b. eggs, liver, rye bread and apples
    c. eggs, liver, apples, and carrots
    d. eggs, liver, spinach, and carrots

68. A 25-year-old woman has a 35 mg. daily intake of ascorbic acid. Compared with the RDA for this age group her intake is

    a. 100% adequate
    b. 75% adequate
    c. 50% adequate
    d. 33% adequate

69. The vitamins taken in excess over a prolonged period of time which can produce hypervitaminosis are

    A. vitamin A
    B. riboflavin
    C. thiamine
    D. vitamin D

    a. A and B
    b. B and C
    c. C and D
    d. A and D

70. The vitamin which is measured in I.U. (International Units) is

    a. thiamine
    b. vitamin K
    c. vitamin D
    d. folic acid

71. The amount of vitamin D that has to be added to milk under the enrichment law is

    a. 4,000 I.U.
    b. 5,000 I.U.
    c. 400 I.U.
    d. 500 I.U.

72. The amount of vitamin D that has to be added to oleomargarine under the enrichment law is no less than

    a. 15,000 I.U. per ounce
    b. 15,000 I.U. per pound
    c. 15,000 I.U. per gram
    d. 15,000 I.U. per cup

73. Vitamin D aids in the absorption of the mineral

    a. iron
    b. fluorine
    c. iodine
    d. calcium

74. Which of the following foods are good sources of folic acid?

    A. cauliflower
    B. spinach
    C. rice
    D. yeast

    a. A and B
    b. B and D
    c. C and D
    d. all of the above

75. The vitamin necessary for the regeneration of red blood cells is

    a. thiamine
    b. folic acid
    c. pantothenic acid
    d. vitamin A

76. The vitamin also called "Castle's extrinsic factor" is

    a. cyanocobalamin
    b. folic acid
    c. pantothenic acid
    d. riboflavin

77. For the human body to convert folic acid into a biologically active form, the substances required are

    A. B_{12}
    B. pantothenic acid
    C. ascorbic acid
    D. niacin

    a. A and B
    b. A and C
    c. A and D
    d. none of the above

78. The anti-vitamin K substance is

    a. menadione
    b. Dicumarol
    c. dehydrocholesterol
    d. glucose

79. Substances for which Recommended Dietary Allowances have not been established are

    A. vitamin A
    B. vitamin E
    C. ascorbic acid
    D. choline

    a. A and D
    b. B and C
    c. B and D
    d. A and C

80. For which of the following functions is vitamin B_6 needed?

    A. decarboxylation
    B. regeneration of red blood cells
    C. blood clotting
    D. transamination

    a. A and B
    b. A and C
    c. A and D
    d. all of the above

81. Insulin, a hormone, is needed by the body to

    a. convert fatty acids to neutral fats
    b. convert glucose to glycogen
    c. convert glycogen to glucose
    d. convert glucose to fructose

82. Compared to fresh whole milk, skim milk contains less

    a. calories, vitamin C, and calcium
    b. calories, vitamin A, and ascorbic acid
    c. calories, vitamin A, and vitamin D
    d. calories, vitamin A, and fat

83. The water content of fresh cow's milk is approximately

    a. 50% of the total weight
    b. 60% of the total weight
    c. 75% of the total weight
    d. 90% of the total weight

84. If your daily food intake contained 250 calories above your energy requirement, you might gain in four weeks

    a. 1 pound
    b. 1½ pounds
    c. 2 pounds
    d. 2½ pounds

85. Of the following foods, those containing empty calories are

    A. granulated sugar
    B. grapefruit
    C. carbonated beverages
    D. cabbage

    a. A and B
    b. A and C
    c. A and D
    d. all of the above

86. The most economical form of food energy is found in

    a. cereals
    b. potato
    c. cottage cheese
    d. margarine

87. The outstanding nutritional contributions of eggs are

    a. calcium, riboflavin, and vitamin K
    b. calcium, iron, and protein
    c. calcium, riboflavin, and protein
    d. calcium, ascorbic acid, and protein

88. Which of the following nutrients are considered to be cariogenic?

    a. protein, starch, and sucrose
    b. sucrose, glucose, and starch
    c. phosphorus, calcium, and fluorine
    d. sulphur, iron, and magnesium

89. Of the following foods, which ones contain only complete proteins?

    a. milk and gelatin
    b. enriched white bread and cheese
    c. milk and American cheese
    d. navy beans and frankfurter

90. Compared to that for middle aged adults, the thiamine requirement of the older person is

    a. higher
    b. lower
    c. the same
    d. dependent on the protein in the diet

91. Gingivitis can frequently result from a nutrient deficiency in

    a. vitamin A
    b. riboflavin
    c. ascorbic acid
    d. phosphorus

92. Co-carboxylase is needed in the human body for the purpose of

    a. breaking down of fats to fatty acids and glycerol
    b. transporting of fats in the lymph
    c. energy production
    d. transamination

93. A condition that prevails in many areas of the world because of poor protein intake is

    a. goiter
    b. kwashiorkor
    c. night blindness
    d. scurvy

94. An example of mutual supplementation of proteins is

    a. corn and gelatin
    b. corn and lysine
    c. corn and beans
    d. corn and milk

95. Which one of the following nutrients is known as an antioxidant?

    a. vitamin K
    b. vitamin E
    c. vitamin D
    d. vitamin B_{12}

96. Of the following substances, which ones are acted upon by the enzyme trypsin?

    a. glucose and glycerol
    b. protein and starch
    c. peptones and peptides
    d. glucose and peptides

97. A substance that is synthesized to cholesterol in the human body is called

    a. glucose
    b. squalene
    c. chilomicron
    d. acetone

98. A woman 25-year-old weighs 50 kg. Her total diet contains 33 gm. proteins. Compared to the protein recommendations for her age group this is

    a. ⅔ of the Recommended Daily Dietary Allowance
    b. ½ of the Recommended Daily Dietary Allowance
    c. ⅓ of the Recommended Daily Dietary Allowance
    d. ¼ of the Recommended Daily Dietary Allowance

99. The correct sequence of the formula to be used for the determination of total energy metabolism is

    a. SDA + cost of activities + BMR
    b. BMR + SDA + cost of activities
    c. cost of activities + SDA + BMR
    d. BMR + cost of activities + SDA

100. A person has a total energy requirement of 2950 calories daily. His basal metabolic rate is 1400 calories. The SDA (Specific Dynamic Action) is 270 calories. The energy cost of his activities is covered by

    a. 1,100 calories
    b. 1,200 calories
    c. 1,300 calories
    d. 1,400 calories

ANSWERS

1. b	26. a	51. a	76. a
2. d	27. d	52. c	77. b
3. c	28. c	53. c	78. b
4. b	29. c	54. a	79. c
5. c	30. b	55. c	80. c
6. c	31. c	56. a	81. b
7. a	32. c	57. c	82. d
8. a	33. c	58. d	83. d
9. c	34. a	59. b	84. c
10. a	35. b	60. a	85. b
11. c	36. a	61. a	86. a
12. d	37. d	62. c	87. b
13. d	38. a	63. c	88. b
14. b	39. c	64. b	89. c
15. c	40. b	65. c	90. b
16. b	41. d	66. a	91. c
17. c	42. b	67. d	92. c
18. b	43. d	68. c	93. b
19. b	44. c	69. d	94. c
20. d	45. c	70. c	95. b
21. b	46. d	71. c	96. c
22. b	47. b	72. b	97. b
23. b	48. a	73. d	98. a
24. b	49. a	74. b	99. d
25. c	50. b	75. b	100. c

REFERENCES

1. Bogert, L. J., Briggs, G. M., and Calloway, D. H.: *Nutrition and Physical Fitness.* 8th Ed. Philadelphia, W. B. Saunders, 1966.
2. Proudfit, F. K., and Robinson, C. H.: *Normal and Therapeutic Nutrition.* 13th Ed. New York, Macmillan Co., 1967.

CHAPTER 9

CLINICAL DENTAL HYGIENE

Ruth R. Swords

1. On the first appointment with a patient whose case requires multiple appointments, the dental hygienist should strive to accomplish which of the following lists of objectives?

    a. establishment of rapport with the patient, preparation of records, removal of gross deposits from teeth, and instruction of the patient in proper methods of home care

    b. establishment of rapport with the patient, preparation of records, application of fluorides topically to the teeth, and instruction of the patient in proper methods of home care

    c. preparation of records, removal of gross deposits from teeth, polishing of teeth, and instruction of the patient in proper methods of home care

    d. preparation of records, removal of gross deposits from teeth, polishing of teeth, and application of fluorides topically to the teeth

2. The best time of day for dental appointments with pre-school children is in the

    a. mid-morning

    b. early afternoon

    c. mid-afternoon

    d. late afternoon

3. Appointments that are made as much as two weeks in advance are often broken because the patients forget them. The *best* way to prevent an appointment from being broken because it is forgotten is

    a. to explain to the patient what a tremendous loss a broken appointment represents to him as well as to you

    b. to have the patient repeat to you the date, day, and time of the appointment at the time you make it

    c. to give the patient a card on which the date, day, and time of the appointment have been noted

    d. to remind the patient by mail or by telephone the day before the appointment

4. Of the outline drawings shown below, which one illustrates correct position in the dental chair?

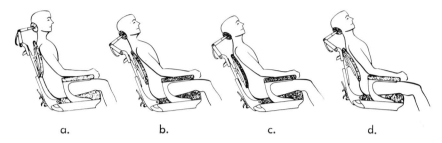

a.   b.   c.   d.

5. When a patient is received and seated in the dental chair, which of the following situations impresses him most favorably?

   a. The instrument tray has not yet been cleared of instruments used on the preceding patient, and this task is performed as the patient watches.
   b. The instrument tray has been cleared of instruments used on the preceding patient, but the tray cover and cup for water have not yet been changed.
   c. The instrument tray has been cleared of instruments, and the cover and cup used by the preceding patient have been discarded. As the patient watches, a fresh tray cover and cup are put in place, and instruments needed for his work are taken from their sanitized storage area and put in place on the tray.
   d. Instruments that will be needed for this patient's work are already in place on the instrument tray. The cup is in its place and already filled with water.

6. When a patient's head is positioned correctly and the mouth is opened comfortably, the lines of the occlusal surfaces of the maxillary teeth and the mandibular teeth will form angles with a horizontal plane, respectively, of

   a. 60 degrees and 45 degrees
   b. 45 degrees and 15 degrees
   c. 30 degrees and 0 degrees
   d. 15 degrees and −15 degrees

7. The backrest of the dental chair should be adjusted to support which area of the patient's back?

   a. cervicothoracic
   b. thoracic
   c. lumbar
   d. lumbosacral

8. Maximum illumination of the dental arches generally is achieved by adjusting the light in accordance with which of the following procedures?

   a. Raise the light to produce a downward beam for the upper arch and lower the light to produce an upward beam for the lower arch.
   b. Lower the light to produce an upward beam for the upper arch and raise the light to produce a downward beam for the lower arch.
   c. Place the light so that the beam will be parallel to the dental arch to be illuminated.
   d. Adjust the light so that the beam and a horizontal plane form an angle of 85 degrees for both arches.

9. When the dental hygienist wishes to use a pamphlet which gives detailed instruction on some facet of home care for the patient, which of the following methods of presentation will be most effective?

   a. The pamphlet is given to the patient when he arrives so that it can be read before the patient is seated in the dental chair.
   b. The pamphlet is given to the patient at the time of chairside instruction, but the material covered in the pamphlet will not be included in the instruction.
   c. The material covered in the pamphlet is explained during chairside instruction, and important points are underlined in the patient's presence.
   d. The pamphlet is mailed to the patient so that it can be read at the patient's leisure.

10. In training a child to brush his teeth properly, which of the following procedures should the dental hygienist employ?

   a. Only the child should be educated because he is more receptive to instruction.
   b. Only the parent should be educated because he has a longer attention span.
   c. Both the parent and the child should be educated so that any limiting factor in the learning process may be overcome.
   d. It is necessary to educate not only the child but both parents if the instruction is to be successful.

11. What is the optimal time in which teeth should be brushed after eating?

   a. within the first ten minutes after eating
   b. within the first thirty minutes after eating
   c. within the first hour after eating
   d. within one to two hours after eating

12. In learning the proper way to brush his teeth, the patient gains most

    a. from a verbal explanation of how it should be done
    b. from observing a demonstration on a model of how it should be done
    c. by demonstrating on a model, following the hygienist's instructions
    d. by demonstrating in his own mouth with a toothbrush, following the hygienist's instructions

13. Which of the following concepts should guide the dental hygienist when she is engaged in patient education?

    A. Patients can be expected to master a simple new home care technique after one period of instruction.
    B. Many patients will need at least two sessions of instruction to master even the simplest new home care technique.
    C. Mastery of a complex home care technique will require many sessions of instruction.
    D. All patients need review and reinstruction periodically.

    a. A, C, and D
    b. B, C, and D
    c. A and D
    d. B and D

14. Which one of the following toothbrushing techniques is most likely to clean the gingival sulcus?

    a. rolling stroke method
    b. modified Stillman's method
    c. Bass' method
    d. Charters' method

15. Which of the following list of dimensions is recommended by the Council on Dental Therapeutics for the brushing surface of a toothbrush designed for general *adult* use?

    a. $\frac{3}{4}$ to $1\frac{1}{2}$ inches long by $\frac{1}{4}$ to $\frac{1}{2}$ inches wide
    b. 1 to $1\frac{1}{4}$ inches long by $\frac{5}{16}$ to $\frac{3}{8}$ inches wide
    c. 1 to $1\frac{1}{2}$ inches long by $\frac{1}{4}$ to $\frac{3}{8}$ inches wide
    d. $1\frac{1}{2}$ to $1\frac{3}{4}$ inches long by $\frac{5}{16}$ to $\frac{3}{8}$ inches wide

16. Which one of the following would be *contraindicated* as an ingredient for a dentifrice?

    a. essential oil
    b. polysaccharide
    c. abrasive
    d. binding agent

17. A solution of ½ teaspoon of table salt in 8 ounces of water has an osmotic pressure with the oral tissue fluids which is

    a. hypotonic
    b. isotonic
    c. mildly hypertonic
    d. extremely hypertonic

18. Mouthwash manufacturers claim their products have beneficial germicidal effects. Which of the following statements concerning this effect is true?

    a. Germicidal effects have been proved in test tubes.
    b. Clinical and laboratory results have been proved comparable.
    c. A nonspecific change in normal oral flora has been proved beneficial.
    d. Oral microorganisms, per se, have been proved to be the primary etiologic factor in oral disease.

19. A soothing and healing rinse recommended for use following extensive instrumentation is a solution of table salt in which of the following proportions?

    a. ½ tsp. salt in 8 oz. of warm water
    b. ¾ tsp. salt in 8 oz. of warm water
    c. 1 tsp. salt in 8 oz. of warm water
    d. 1½ tsp. salt in 8 oz. of warm water

20. Which of the following are desired objectives of gingival massage?

    A. promotion of keratinization
    B. promotion of passive hyperemia
    C. stimulation of circulation
    D. decrease in sensitivity

    a. A, B, and D
    b. A, C, and D
    c. A and C
    d. all of the above

21. Following is a list of procedures. Which of these is *not* a recommended procedure for the dental hygienist to carry out when she dismisses a patient?

    a. Clean the patient's face of any stain or debris.

    b. Lower the chair and clear the patient's path of any obstacle.

    c. Explain to the patient how the recall system works and how he will be notified if he wishes to be reminded when it is time to return to the dental office.

    d. Suggest that the patient learn as much as he can about oral home care from the educational media at his disposal, television, radio, newspapers, and magazines.

22. The dentist and the patient's physician should be consulted before the appointment for an oral prophylaxis for a patient taking an anticoagulant because patients taking anticoagulants are predisposed to

    a. vasomotor instability

    b. phlebothrombosis

    c. neurogenic shock

    d. capillary hemorrhage

23. A history of rheumatic fever in a patient who is to receive an oral prophylaxis is a matter of concern to the dental hygienist because rheumatic fever predisposes the patient to

    a. coronary occlusion

    b. pulmonary thrombosis

    c. subacute bacterial endocarditis

    d. myocardial infarction

24. While making the oral inspection, the dental hygienist notices a small, circumscribed, elevated, translucent, bluish lesion on the mucosa of the lower lip. The patient gives a history of previous experience with other such lesions at the same site which have ruptured, discharged a sticky material, and collapsed. When the area seemingly has healed, the lesion has recurred. This cycle has been repeated for weeks. The lesion is most likely to be diagnosed by the dentist as a

    a. ranula

    b. mucocele

    c. sialolith

    d. multilocular cyst

25. Charting of the patient's mouth should optimally be done in what sequence with other procedures of the appointment?

    a. before the prophylaxis
    b. following the prophylaxis but preceding the fluoride treatment
    c. following the prophylaxis and fluoride treatment
    d. following the prophylaxis, fluoride treatment, and chairside in-
       struction

26. The two types of chart forms commonly used in dental offices are

    a. anatomic and geometric
    b. anatomic and odontic
    c. anatomic and isometric
    d. odontic and geometric

27. In interpreting a roentgenogram in which a deposit of calculus is plainly visible on the interproximal surface of a tooth, one may assume that the depth of the pocket at that point will be at what level?

    a. exactly at the level of the apical end of the deposit
    b. a millimeter or so below the apical end of the deposit
    c. four or five millimeters below the apical end of the deposit
    d. a millimeter or so occlusal to the apical end of the deposit

28. While charting the dentition of a child, the dental hygienist finds the following teeth present in all four quadrants of the mouth:
        permanent central incisor
        permanent lateral incisor
        deciduous cuspid (primary canine)
        deciduous first molar (primary first molar)
        deciduous second molar (primary second molar)
        permanent first molar
This eruptive pattern may be considered most nearly normal for a child aged

    a. 3 to 6 years
    b. 7 to 10 years
    c. 11 to 14 years
    d. 15 to 18 years

29. When charting the existing conditions that she finds in a patient's mouth, the dental hygienist may record a possible *distoclusion* when

  a. the mesiobuccal cusp of the maxillary first permanent molar occludes with the buccal groove of the mandibular first permanent molar
  b. the buccal groove of the mandibular first permanent molar is distal to the mesiobuccal cusp of the maxillary first permanent molar by at least the width of a bicuspid
  c. the buccal groove of the mandibular first permanent molar is mesial to the mesiobuccal cusp of the maxillary first permanent molar by at least the width of a bicuspid
  d. the mesiobuccal cusp of the maxillary first permanent molar is distal to the buccal groove of the mandibular first permanent molar by at least the width of a bicuspid

30. A young patient tells the dental hygienist that she has a long-standing habit of sucking lemons. The patient has loss of tooth substance affecting the anterior teeth. The gradual loss of tooth substance which has occurred in this case is most likely to be appropriately noted on the chart as

  a. attrition
  b. erosion
  c. abrasion
  d. intrusion

31. The dentist has noted on the patient's chart that the gingival tissue in a specified area is *edematous*. To which of the following conditions does this term refer?

  a. The capillaries of the area are congested due to increased inflow of blood.
  b. The capillaries of the area are congested due to decreased outflow of blood.
  c. An abnormally large amount of fluid is present in the intercellular tissue spaces of the area.
  d. An abnormally large amount of fluid is present in the tissue cells of the area.

32. When the dental hygienist notices that the patient has white or yellowish granules on the buccal mucosa at the level of the occlusal plane of the teeth, this finding should be noted on the patient's record. The dentist's diagnosis of this condition would most likely be

  a. Addison's disease
  b. Fordyce disease
  c. Paget's disease
  d. Mikulicz's disease

33. Which chart represents the correct record of existing conditions in the mouth of a patient who has the following missing teeth and restorations?

UR8 missing

UR6 MOD amalgam

UR3 ¾ gold crown

UR2 missing (pontic of bridge)

UR1 ¾ gold crown

UR3-X-UR1 (fixed prosthesis)

UL1 mesial silicate

UL7 MO amalgam

UL8 missing

LR8 missing (radiograph shows impaction)

LR7 MOD amalgam

LL6 MOD gold inlay

LL7 MO gold inlay

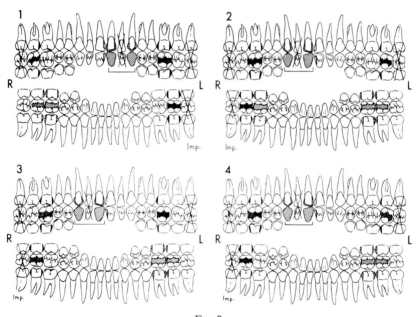

FIG. 9

Chart Code:

Missing teeth	= Marked X
Amalgam restorations	= Filled in
Gold restorations	= Diagonal lines used
Synthetic restorations	= Blank
Removable prosthesis	= Bracket above teeth
Fixed prosthesis	= Bracket below teeth

a. chart number one

b. chart number two

c. chart number three

d. chart number four

34. A patient who has requested an appointment to have his teeth cleaned is seated in the chair and the dental hygienist begins the oral inspection. She notices the patient has an offensive mouth odor, highly inflamed gingivae, and blunted interdental papillae covered with a yellowish gray membrane. When the membrane is removed with an explorer, the tissue is denuded and bleeds copiously. The patient gives a history of a sudden onset of pain which has prevented his brushing his teeth and has even interfered with his eating. The dental hygienist should ask the dentist to examine the patient immediately for she knows the dentist will find the signs and symptoms in this patient to be diagnostic of

   a. stomatitis medicamentosa
   b. herpangina
   c. erosive lichen planus
   d. necrotizing ulcerative gingivitis

35. Of the following list of enamel hypoplasias, which one is hereditary?

   a. dental fluorosis
   b. systemic hypoplasia
   c. local hypoplasia
   d. amelogenesis imperfecta

36. Which of the following would *not* be considered an anatomic limitation to proper use of a toothbrush?

   a. narrow arch
   b. short lingual frenum
   c. taut musculature of cheeks and lips
   d. microglossia

37. Which of the following alterations in the gingivae and the teeth may be attributed to toothbrush trauma?

   A. notched and grooved gingivae
   B. McCall's festoons
   C. wedge-shaped concavities in facial surfaces of teeth
   D. gingival hyperplasia

   a. B and C
   b. A, B, and C
   c. B, C, and D
   d. all of the above

38. Which of the following diagnostic aids is *least* valuable to the dentist in the diagnosis of periodontal pockets?

   a. periodontal probe
   b. mouth mirror
   c. radiographs
   d. study models

39. When the oral inspection reveals gingival enlargement which is *not* associated with primary inflammation, the condition is most likely to be associated with

    a. pregnancy
    b. leukemia
    c. vitamin C deficiency
    d. Dilantin therapy

40. During the oral inspection the dental hygienist notices that the patient's entire tongue is abnormally red, smooth, and shiny. The patient complains of burning and numbness of the tongue, sensitivity to hot and spicy foods, and pain on swallowing. There is marked pallor of the gingiva. All these findings will be recorded on the patient's chart for the dentist's attention. During his examination he will most likely associate these findings with which of the following diseases?

    a. stomatitis medicamentosa
    b. scarlet fever
    c. glossitis areata migrans
    d. pernicious anemia

41. During the oral inspection the dental hygienist notices an irregular, white, necrotic lesion in the soft tissue surrounding an impacted third molar. When the patient is questioned concerning the duration of the lesion, he states that it developed during the night immediately preceding the appointment. It is also learned that the development of the lesion was preceded by pain which he had attempted to relieve by self-medication. This condition is most likely to be diagnosed by the dentist as

    a. stomatitis medicamentosa
    b. nicotinic stomatitis
    c. moniliasis
    d. aspirin burn

42. According to recent findings, which one of the following is *not* essential to formation of calculus?

    a. increase in pH
    b. saliva
    c. bacteria
    d. mucopolysaccharides

43. There are several ways in which calculus is attached by its bacterial matrix to tooth surfaces. Calculus deposits most readily removed are those attached by which of the following modes of adherence?

    a. to the secondary cuticle
    b. to minute irregularities in the surface of the cementum or enamel
    c. to cementum by penetration to various depths
    d. to cementum by penetration into areas of cemental resorption

44. Which of the following is *not* a predisposing factor in the formation of dental plaque?

    a. natural tendencies of the individual
    b. thick mucinous saliva which stagnates around the teeth
    c. oral flora
    d. high pH of saliva

45. Of the following abnormal conditions that affect both morphology and tooth crown color, which can be prevented most easily by alert medical and dental practitioners?

    a. fluorescent yellow stain
    b. fluorosis
    c. amelogenesis imperfecta
    d. dentinogenesis imperfecta

46. Of the following stains, which occurs frequently in a clean mouth?

    a. yellow stain
    b. green stain
    c. black stain
    d. orange and red stains

47. Which one of the following stains is *not* extrinsic?

    a. black line stain
    b. green stain
    c. fluorescent yellow stain
    d. tobacco stain

48. Which stain can be classified as exogenous intrinsic?

    a. fluorescent yellow stain
    b. black stain
    c. green stain
    d. ammoniacal silver nitrate stain

49. The dental hygienist will probably find the largest deposits of calculus on the

    a. lingual surfaces of the upper incisors and the buccal surfaces of the lower molars

    b. lingual surfaces of the lower incisors and the buccal surfaces of the upper molars

    c. labial surfaces of the lower incisors and the lingual surfaces of the upper molars

    d. labial surfaces of the upper incisors and the lingual surfaces of the upper molars

50. The removal of green stain from enamel is facilitated by the application of which of the following disclosing solutions prior to polishing?

    a. basic fuchsin

    b. iodine

    c. Bismarck brown

    d. mercurochrome

51. A balanced instrument is one that

    a. will maintain equilibrium when it is held so that it may pivot on the end of the index finger

    b. is double-ended, having blades on each end

    c. has a blade that is centered along the long axis of the handle

    d. has a hollow handle

52. The concave or magnifying mirror's chief advantage over the plane mirror is that

    a. it gives a more distinct and larger image

    b. it concentrates rays of light and therefore illuminates some areas of the mouth better than the plane mirror

    c. its concave surface is more comfortable to soft tissue when used for retraction

    d. it maintains a clear reflecting surface longer than the plane mirror when subjected to regular autoclaving

53. The mouth mirror should *not* be used

    a. to make visible those areas of the mouth that cannot be seen by direct vision

    b. to reflect light so that obscure areas may be properly illuminated

    c. as a fulcrum during any of the prophylactic procedures

    d. to retract soft tissue in order to have more accessibility to the area being instrumented

54. The type of mirror that is *contraindicated* for use in a dental examination is the

    a. plane mirror
    b. magnifying mirror
    c. front surface mirror
    d. fluorescent mirror

55. Which of the following procedures are recommended to prevent "fogging" of mouth mirrors?

    A. Wipe the mirror with an alcohol sponge.
    B. Warm the mirror by placing it in warm water.
    C. Ask the patient to breathe through his nose.
    D. Wipe the mirror against the patient's buccal mucosa.

    a. A, B, and C
    b. A, C, and D
    c. B, C, and D
    d. all of the above

56. Which of the following is *not* a recommended use for an explorer?

    a. detection of tooth hyposensitivity
    b. detection of irregularities of tooth surfaces
    c. detection of calculus deposits
    d. detection of carious lesions

57. When an explorer is used near or under the gingival margin, the angle that the working end makes with the tooth surface should fall within the range of

    a. 75 to 90 degrees
    b. 50 to 65 degrees
    c. 30 to 45 degrees
    d. 5 to 20 degrees

58. Which of the following is *not* an expected result of maintaining a sharp explorer tip?

    a. more tactile sensitivity
    b. decreased operating time
    c. increased patient comfort
    d. increased likelihood of unnecessary gingival trauma

59. Which of the following techniques is *incorrect* for use of the periodontal probe?

    a. use pen grasp of instrument and a stable fulcrum
    b. insert blade gently but firmly into the sulcus until tissue resistance is felt
    c. hold blade perpendicular to long axis of tooth during application
    d. identify depth of pocket by checking millimeter marks on blade

60. The facial surface of the blade of the curet should be positioned so that it forms with the tooth surface an angle of

   a. slightly less than 80 degrees
   b. slightly less than 85 degrees
   c. slightly less than 90 degrees
   d. slightly more than 95 degrees

61. The cross-section view of the blade of the curet is that of

   a. an isosceles triangle
   b. a trapezoid
   c. a crescent
   d. an ellipse

62. Which one of the following instruments usually is used for finishing the scaling phase of the oral prophylaxis?

   a. sickle
   b. curet
   c. hoe
   d. chisel

63. Which instrument can be considered to have one continuous cutting edge?

   a. sickle
   b. curet
   c. hoe
   d. chisel

64. Which one of the instruments listed below is versatile enough to be used to accomplish all of the following: removal of necrotic cementum; removal of submarginal calculus, particularly deposits which are located deep within the pocket; removal of small deposits of supramarginal calculus which adhere after gross deposits have been removed; and production of a smooth root surface through root planing?

   a. sickle
   b. curet
   c. hoe
   d. chisel

65. The jacquette scaler is classified as a

   a. sickle
   b. curet
   c. hoe
   d. chisel

66. Of the outline drawings shown below, which one illustrates correct positioning of the blade of the sickle scaler to the tooth surface?

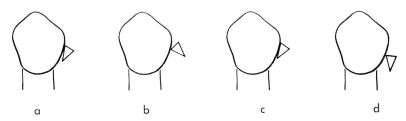

a   b   c   d

67. Of the outline drawings shown below, which one illustrates correct positioning of the curet scaler to the tooth surface?

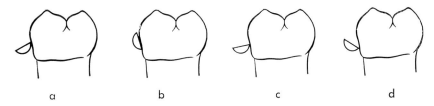

a   b   c   d

68. Of the outline drawings shown below, which one illustrates correct position of the hoe scaler on the tooth surface?

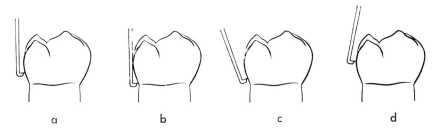

a   b   c   d

69. During activation of a scaling instrument, the facial surface of the blade and the tooth surface should form an angle of

   a. more than 90 degrees but less than 180 degrees
   b. more than 30 degrees but less than 60 degrees
   c. more than 45 degrees but less than 90 degrees
   d. more than 15 degrees but less than 45 degrees

70. What determines the areas and tooth surfaces to which a sickle scaler can be applied?

   a. angulation and flexibility of the blade
   b. angulation and flexibility of the shank
   c. angulation and length of the blade
   d. angulation and length of the shank

71. The sickle scaler is used primarily for

    a. root planing

    b. removing heavy deposits of calculus located supramarginally or submarginally only to a slight depth

    c. removing granular calculus from smooth surfaces of the teeth

    d. removing heavy deposits of calculus located supramarginally or submarginally to the depth of the periodontal pocket (including depths of more than 3 millimeters)

72. The direction of the stroke used in scaling teeth is determined by

    a. the pattern of distribution of the deposits on the teeth being scaled

    b. the position of the tooth being scaled, since the direction of the stroke must be parallel to the long axis of the tooth

    c. those factors that contribute to maximum comfort for the patient

    d. the instrument, the area of the mouth, and the tooth surface to which the instrument is applied

73. When an instrument is activated in what is referred to as the *working* stroke, in which of the following ways is it employed?

    a. The instrument is pushed gently toward the gingiva.

    b. Pressure is exerted as the instrument is pulled away from the epithelial attachment and gingiva.

    c. The instrument is directed so that the force of the stroke is perpendicular to the long axis of the tooth.

    d. The instrument is pushed to the depth of the sulcus to engage the calculus.

74. The three phases of the scaling stroke in proper sequence, are

    a. application, angulation, activation

    b. angulation, application, activation

    c. activation, angulation, application

    d. application, activation, angulation

75. When ultrasonic vibration is used in periodontal instrumentation, the frequency at which the tip is vibrated is approximately

    a. 25,000 cycles per second

    b. 50,000 cycles per second

    c. 75,000 cycles per second

    d. 100,000 cycles per second

76. According to current research, the major advantage of ultrasonic scaling techniques is in

    a. removal of stain
    b. removal of supramarginal calculus
    c. removal of gross calculus deposits, both submarginal and supra-marginal
    d. removal of both stain and calculus so rapidly and so efficiently that hand instrumentation is not necessary

77. Which of the following list of advantages does the soft polishing cup have over the hard polishing cup?

    A. more flexible
    B. less likely to abrade soft tissue
    C. more efficient in removing soft deposits and stains
    D. more easily adapted to relatively inaccessible tooth surfaces

    a. A only
    b. A and D
    c. A, B, and D
    d. all of the above

78. Of the following, which is *inversely* proportional to the rapidity of abrasion?

    a. the number of particles applied per unit of time
    b. the speed of application
    c. the pressure applied
    d. the amount of liquid added to the abrasive agent

79. The coarsest abrasive suitable for use on tooth surfaces is

    a. F flour of pumice
    b. FF flour of pumice
    c. FFF flour of pumice
    d. FFFF flour of pumice

80. Why should dry polishing powders or flours be mixed with a liquid before they are applied to the tooth surface?

    a. Wetting the polishing agent causes more particles of the agent to reach the surface being polished per unit of time.
    b. Wetting the polishing agent increases the rate of abrasion.
    c. Wetting the polishing agent reduces frictional heat.
    d. Wetting the polishing agent causes a chemical change which facilitates the polishing.

81. When abrasive strips are employed to remove small pieces of supra-marginal calculus and extrinsic stains, their use should be limited to the

    a. facial surfaces of the teeth
    b. lingual surfaces of the teeth
    c. proximal surfaces of the teeth, incisal or occlusal to the interdental soft tissue
    d. proximal surfaces of the teeth, from depth of sulcus to incisal or occlusal

82. Which one of the following grades of cuttle or abrasive strip is appropriate for dental hygiene techniques?

    a. coarse grade
    b. medium grade
    c. fine grade
    d. extra fine grade

83. Which one of the following methods of using dental floss is correct?

    a. The floss is snapped through the contact.
    b. The floss is held parallel to the occlusal surfaces of the teeth.
    c. A short grasp of the floss is maintained throughout its use.
    d. Floss is removed by pulling it through the embrasure against the papilla.

84. The most commonly used agent for cleansing the proximal surfaces of the teeth is dental floss or tape. Which of the following agents also are recommended to be used for this purpose?

    A. three-ply nylon or rayon knitting yarn
    B. three-ply wool knitting yarn
    C. gauze strips
    D. rubber, wood, or plastic interdental stimulators

    a. A, B, and C
    b. A, C, and D
    c. D only
    d. all of the above

85. For cleaning an acrylic denture, which of the following procedures is *contraindicated?*

    a. Protect the denture from breakage by preparing a cushion to receive it in case it should be dropped.
    b. Grasp the denture firmly in the palm of the hand while cleaning it.
    c. Place the denture in a mild chemical solution.
    d. Rinse the denture under a moderate stream of hot water.

86. Which of the following is *not* recommended for use as a denture cleaner?

    a. toilet soap
    b. bicarbonate of soda
    c. precipitated calcium carbonate
    d. scouring abrasive

87. A solution of white vinegar is recommended as a cleansing agent for dentures. To make a solution to be used for this purpose, the operator should add to 1 cup of water

    a. 1 tsp. vinegar
    b. 1 tbsp. vinegar
    c. $\frac{1}{4}$ c. vinegar
    d. $\frac{1}{2}$ c. vinegar

88. Which one of the following agents should be used to polish amalgam restorations?

    a. tin oxide
    b. zinc oxide
    c. mercuric oxide
    d. cupric oxide

89. Which of the following agents should be used for visual evaluation of the oral prophylaxis?

    A. compressed air
    B. transilluminator
    C. disclosing solution
    D. explorer

    a. A and C
    b. A, B, and C
    c. B, C, and D
    d. all of the above

90. The most objective method for evaluating the completeness of oral prophylaxis is

    a. transillumination
    b. radiographs
    c. compressed air
    d. tactile sensation

91. Which of the following are contraindications for the use of air under pressure as a means of checking the proficiency of the oral prophylaxis?

    A. silicate restorations
    B. gold restorations
    C. hypersensitive dentition
    D. dental caries

    a. A only
    b. A and B
    c. A, C, and D
    d. all of above

92. A history of diabetes *contraindicates* the use of disclosing agents that contain

    a. erythrosin dye
    b. basic fuchsin
    c. iodine
    d. mercurochrome

93. For a patient who has synthetic restorations, the preferred disclosing agent should contain

    a. erythrosin dye
    b. iodine
    c. mercurochrome
    d. Bismarck brown

94. A patient has always lived in an area where the water supply contained the optimal amount of fluoride, yet this patient shows evidence of caries. Would topical application of fluoride be indicated? Why?

    a. Yes, because research has shown that there is an additive effect when the patient receives both ingested and topical fluorides.
    b. No, because the enamel already has received as much benefit as it can from the ingested fluoride.
    c. No, because the use of topical fluorides in addition to the ingested fluorides might cause fluorosis.
    d. No, because the presence of caries in this patient shows that the enamel of his teeth does not receive benefit from fluoride.

95. Topically applied fluorides penetrate into sound tooth enamel to a depth of

    a. .001 mm.
    b. .01 mm.
    c. 0.1 mm.
    d. 1.0 mm.

96. Recent clinical studies have indicated that topical application of sodium fluoride solutions acidified with orthophosphoric acid produces

    a. an increase in caries incidence
    b. no reduction in caries incidence
    c. some reduction in caries incidence, but not enough to be statistically significant
    d. a highly significant reduction in caries incidence

97. Following application of topical fluoride compounds to the teeth of a patient, the dental hygienist should instruct him not to rinse his mouth or ingest anything for a period of

    a. 15 minutes
    b. 30 minutes
    c. 45 minutes
    d. 60 minutes

98. Which of the following items should *not* be used prior to the application of topical fluoride compounds?

    a. dental floss or tape made of silk
    b. dental floss or tape made of nylon
    c. dental floss or tape that is waxed
    d. dental floss or tape that is unwaxed

99. Which of the following is the correct procedure to follow if saliva enters the isolated field and wets the tooth surfaces during the topical application of a solution of fluoride?

    a. Take out the cotton rolls used to isolate the teeth and start over.
    b. Wipe off the saliva with gauze and continue the treatment.
    c. Increase the length of time the teeth are kept wet with the fluoride solution.
    d. Continue the treatment without change.

100. For a young patient with decalcified anterior teeth who is leaving town and cannot return to the dental office for a month, which of the following fluoride solutions should be used for topical application?

    a. sodium fluoride solution
    b. stannous fluoride, 8% solution
    c. stannous fluoride, 10% solution
    d. sodium fluoride solution, acidified with orthophosphoric acid

101. The container that is used for storage of sodium fluoride solution should be made of

    a. plain glass
    b. porcelain
    c. polyethylene
    d. metal

102. Cotton rolls that are used to isolate teeth for a topical application of fluoride solution should be cut at a 45 degree angle because

    a. they are more easily placed in the cotton roll holders when beveled in this manner
    b. this is the most convenient way to shorten the cotton roll to the correct length
    c. this increases the cross-sectional area of the most absorbent part of the cotton roll and thereby significantly decreases the chance of wetting the teeth with saliva
    d. beveling the cotton roll facilitates its placement and retention in the proper position

103. Which of the following is *not* a reason for using a topical anesthetic?

    a. low pain threshold
    b. apprehension
    c. hypertension
    d. gagging tendency

104. When sensitivity to para-aminobenzoate anesthetics exists, which of the following topical anesthetics should be used?

    a. butacaine sulfate
    b. benzocaine
    c. naepaine
    d. dyclonine hydrochloride

105. When an antiseptic solution is applied to the gingival papillae (under the direction of the dentist and in accordance with the state law in those states in which this procedure is permitted) which of the following procedures is *not* a part of the recommended technique?

    a. Saturate a small cotton pellet held with cotton pliers in the antiseptic.
    b. Express excess solution.
    c. Retract the lip, cheek, and tongue and apply solution to inter-dental papillae on both facial and lingual surfaces.
    d. Allow patient to rinse.

106. Which of the following antiseptics are recommended for topical application on the oral mucosa?

    A. iodine solution, N.F.
    B. merbromin solution, N.F.
    C. hydrogen peroxide, U.S.P.
    D. phenol, U.S.P.

    a. A only
    b. A and C
    c. A, B, and C
    d. all of the above

107. Which of the following first aid procedures should be carried out for a patient who has syncope?

    A. Place the patient in a recumbent position with his head lower than his feet.
    B. Loosen tight clothing.
    C. Have the patient inhale aromatic spirits of ammonia.
    D. Place a cold pack on the patient's forehead.

    a. A and C
    b. A, B, and C
    c. A, C, and D
    d. all of the above

108. Which of the following agents for evaluating the oral prophylaxis is *contraindicated* for the patient with hypersensitive teeth?

    a. transilluminator
    b. compressed air
    c. disclosing solution
    d. radiograph

109. Which of the following are recommended precautionary measures for the dental hygienist to take when performing an oral prophylaxis for a patient with hypersensitive teeth?

    A. Avoid directing compressed air onto sensitive tooth surfaces.
    B. Provide warm water for rinsing patient's mouth.
    C. Avoid applying instruments directly to sensitive areas, whenever possible.
    D. Apply topical anesthetic to sensitive areas of the teeth.

    a. A only
    b. A and B
    c. A, B, and C
    d. all of above

110. Which one of the following methods of desensitization is particularly adapted to application by the dental hygienist?

    a. fluoride preparations
    b. iontophoresis
    c. albumin precipitants
    d. cavity varnishes

111. In performing an oral prophylaxis for a bedridden patient, which of the following procedures are recommended?

    A. Because of the inconvenience to the patient, plan to finish in one appointment regardless of the challenge presented by the oral condition.
    B. Request that visitors be excluded during the prophylaxis.
    C. Make the appointment seem leisurely so the patient won't feel rushed.
    D. Be sure the patient understands what is being done in each phase of the appointment.

    a. A, B, and C
    b. B, C, and D
    c. A, C, and D
    d. C and D

112. The dental hygienist should use precautionary measures to protect her patient from discomfort when performing an oral prophylaxis for a patient who has

    a. cheilosis
    b. hyperkeratosis
    c. periodontosis
    d. sarcoidosis

113. Avoidance of tissue trauma is of special significance for patients who have

    a. epilepsy
    b. diabetes mellitus
    c. osteoarthritis
    d. periodontitis

114. Which of the following statements regarding the pregnant patient is *not* true?

    a. Short appointments should be planned.
    b. Although the patient will follow her physician's advice concerning diet, certain dietary needs relating to maintenance of oral health should be stressed by the dental hygienist.
    c. Radiography is contraindicated.
    d. Since the patient is subject to abrupt changes in mood, the dental hygienist should adapt her conversation and instruction to the receptiveness of the patient.

115. Hypersensitivity and emotional instability are characteristic of all of the following *except*

    a. diabetes
    b. puberty
    c. menstruation
    d. menopause

116. The aged patient is most likely to choose a

    a. high protein diet
    b. high fat diet
    c. high carbohydrate diet
    d. liquid diet

117. Which of the following is *not* generally characteristic of the aged patient?

    a. lowered basal metabolism
    b. decrease in hearing acuity, especially sensitivity to high tones
    c. increased nearsightedness
    d. decreased glandular secretions

118. Which of the following could most rationally be *omitted* from dental hygiene care for the patient prior to oral surgery?

    a. development of patient rapport
    b. removal of gross deposits of calculus from the teeth
    c. polishing the teeth
    d. instructing the patient in oral care and dietary procedures

119. Of the following list of tests, which one is *not* a dental caries activity test?

    a. Snyder colorimetric test
    b. Aschheim-Zondek test
    c. lactobacillus plate count
    d. reductase test

120. The dental hygienist may use caries activity tests best

    a. as an accurate indication of the caries activitiy of the individual patient
    b. as an accurate indication of the caries susceptibility of the individual patient
    c. as a dramatic indication to the patient that he needs to practice better preventive procedures
    d. as a dramatic indication that the caries process is arrested

121. In the Snyder colorimetric test, the degree of caries susceptibility is signified by

    a. the rapidity with which the test medium changes from yellow to green

    b. the rapidity with which the test medium changes from green to yellow

    c. the rapidity with which the test medium changes from blue to red

    d. the rapidity with which the test medium changes from red to blue

122. In interpreting the results of the lactobacillus plate count, a *moderate* degree of caries activity or susceptibility may be assumed when the number of lactobacilli per milliliter of saliva is

    a. 0 to 1,000

    b. 1,000 to 5,000

    c. 5,000 to 10,000

    d. 10,000 to 50,000

123. Severe curtailment of carbohydrate consumption is generally difficult for which of the following reasons?

    A. Carbohydrates are inexpensive and they are a readily available source of energy.

    B. Psychologically, many people are dependent on the pleasure and satisfaction they derive from consumption of carbohydrates.

    C. Severe curtailment of carbohydrates cannot be achieved without impairing general health.

    D. High protein foods, which are recommended as substitutes for the carbohydrates, are not generally available in this country.

    a. A only

    b. A and B

    c. A, B, and C

    d. all of above

124. Which of the following dietary variables have given consistent *in vitro* animal, clinical, and human experimental evidence of association with caries activity?

    A. The more frequently sugary foods are eaten, the higher the caries activity.

    B. Sugar taken in solid form is more conducive to caries than when taken in a liquid state.

    C. Diets which have sufficient vitamin D are more likely to prevent decay than diets deficient in this vitamin.

    D. The more phosphates added to a cariogenic diet, the less destructive to the teeth will be the sugar.

    a. A only

    b. A and B

    c. A, B, and C

    d. all of above

125. Which of the following lists of methods of sterilization or disinfection is named in order of preference and reliability?

    a. prolonged dry heat, steam under pressure, boiling water, chemical agents

    b. chemical agents, steam under pressure, boiling water, prolonged dry heat

    c. steam under pressure, boiling water, prolonged dry heat, chemical agents

    d. steam under pressure, prolonged dry heat, boiling water, chemical agents

126. The most reliable *sterilizing* agent is

    a. benzalkonium chloride

    b. boiling water

    c. prolonged dry heat

    d. steam under pressure

127. When instruments are to be disinfected through use of a chemical agent, what is the recommended *minimum* period of exposure?

    a. 10 to 20 minutes

    b. 15 to 30 minutes

    c. 30 to 45 minutes

    d. 45 to 60 minutes

128. When using dry heat as a method of sterilization, the operator should use which of the following temperatures and time schedules?

    a. 160° to 180° C (320° to 355° F) for 15 minutes

    b. 160° to 180° C (320° to 355° F) for 30 minutes

    c. 160° to 180° C (320° to 355° F) for 45 minutes

    d. 160° to 180° C (320° to 355° F) for 60 minutes

129. Which of the following lists of sterilizing data is the correct one to follow when using the autoclave?

    a. 121° C, 15 lbs. pressure, 20 minutes

    b. 115° C, 20 lbs. pressure, 10 minutes

    c. 130° C, 10 lbs. pressure, 10 minutes

    d. 100° C, 15 lbs. pressure, 20 minutes

130. Which of the following materials is relatively impervious to steam and is therefore *not* suitable for wrapping articles to be sterilized?

    a. muslin

    b. plastic cloth

    c. paper

    d. gauze

131. The use of a chemical agent for disinfection of instruments is *contraindicated* when the patient on whom they are to be used gives a history of

    a. syphilis
    b. gonorrhea
    c. hepatitis
    d. subacute bacterial endocarditis

132. When a quaternary ammonium compound is to be used as the disinfecting agent, all soap must be carefully rinsed from the articles being prepared for disinfection because any residual soap will cause

    a. deactivation of bactericidal effects, accompanied by conditions which stimulate bacterial growth
    b. reaction with the agent which produces chemicals that have deleterious effects on mucous membranes
    c. reduction in activity of the agent which occurs owing to the presence of alkalies
    d. reaction with the agent which might result in corrosion of any metallic instruments which are disinfected

133. Which of the following agents commonly used for disinfection and/or sterilization are recommended for use on the dental handpiece?

    a. boiling water and hot silicone fluids
    b. hot oil and chemical agents
    c. chemical agents and dry heat
    d. hot oil and steam under pressure

134. Which of the following sharpening stones is natural?

    a. aloxite stone
    b. diamond stone
    c. ruby stone
    d. Arkansas oilstone

135. In general, hand sharpening of instruments with unmounted stones is preferable to sharpening by motor driven mounted stones because

    a. unmounted stones are finer grained
    b. unmounted stones are less likely to change the bevel
    c. unmounted stones wear away less of the instrument surface
    d. unmounted stones are more easily sterilized

136. The edge of the blade of the hoe scaler should be beveled at what angle to the terminal end of the blade?

    a. 100 degrees
    b. 90 degrees
    c. 45 degrees
    d. 15 degrees

137. In testing an instrument for sharpness *visually* one may assume the blade is sharp when

    a. the edge of the blade is bright and shiny
    b. the angle of the face to the lateral surface of the blade appears obtuse
    c. the edge of the blade is a line which does not reflect light
    d. the blade is wire edged

138. The practice of flaming an instrument for short periods of time is an unreliable method of sterilization because

    A. sterilization is probable only if the instrument is brought to red heat
    B. the temper and finish of most dental instruments will be ruined by bringing the instrument to the proper temperature for sterilization
    C. temperatures lower than red heat will not sterilize unless the exposure time is prolonged to the point of making the technique impractical
    D. although the technique may be effective occasionally, it is not consistently effective

    a. B only
    b. A and B
    c. A, B, and C
    d. all of he above

139. Of the following reasons for keeping scaling instruments sharp at all times, which is the most important?

    a. Keeping instruments sharp enables the operator to save time.
    b. Keeping instruments sharp helps to prevent unnecessary trauma and discomfort to the patient.
    c. Keeping instruments sharp will prolong the useful condition of scalers by avoiding the extensive grinding which is necessitated by neglect.
    d. Keeping instruments sharp will help to avoid burnishing the surface of calculus which occurs when a dull blade is drawn across the deposit, thus making the deposit extremely difficult to remove.

140. The pulleys of the engine arm of the dental unit should be lubricated

    a. daily
    b. weekly
    c. biweekly
    d. semiannually

141. After the engine belt has been washed, the proper time to replace it on the pulleys of the engine arm and handpiece is

    a. while it is still wet
    b. as soon as it is dry
    c. after it is dry and has been treated with oil
    d. never, since the engine belt should not be washed

142. In order to dispel odors and clean the drain of the cuspidor of the dental unit, a strong solution of which of the following agents should be poured down the drain once a week?

    a. sodium chloride
    b. sodium fluoride
    c. sodium hydroxide
    d. sodium bicarbonate

143. The dental handpiece should be lubricated

    a. once daily
    b. once weekly
    c. once semimonthly
    d. once monthly

144. The prophylaxis angle *must* be cleaned and lubricated

    a. after each prophylaxis
    b. twice daily
    c. at the end of each day's work
    d. once a week

145. Use of the straight dental handpiece alone is indicated for

    A. intraoral polishing of teeth
    B. intraoral polishing of fixed prostheses
    C. extraoral polishing of removable prostheses
    D. sharpening of instruments

    a. A and B
    b. B and C
    c. C and D
    d. D only

Acknowledgment: I wish to express sincere appreciation to Mr. Edward M. Grube, Professor and Chairman, Department of Visual Education, Baylor University, College of Dentistry. His contribution of preparing these superior drawings has definitely enhanced this chapter.

ANSWERS

1. a	38. d	75. a	112. a
2. a	39. d	76. c	113. b
3. d	40. d	77. c	114. c
4. c	41. d	78. d	115. a
5. c	42. c	79. c	116. c
6. b	43. a	80. c	117. c
7. c	44. d	81. c	118. c
8. b	45. a	82. d	119. b
9. c	46. c	83. c	120. c
10. c	47. c	84. b	121. b
11. a	48. d	85. d	122. c
12. d	49. b	86. d	123. b
13. b	50. b	87. b	124. b
14. c	51. c	88. a	125. d
15. b	52. b	89. b	126. d
16. b	53. c	90. b	127. b
17. c	54. d	91. c	128. d
18. a	55. c	92. c	129. a
19. a	56. a	93. a	130. b
20. b	57. d	94. a	131. c
21. d	58. d	95. c	132. c
22. d	59. c	96. d	133. d
23. c	60. c	97. b	134. d
24. b	61. c	98. c	135. c
25. b	62. b	99. a	136. c
26. a	63. b	100. d	137. c
27. b	64. b	101. c	138. d
28. b	65. a	102. d	139. d
29. b	66. d	103. c	140. b
30. b	67. d	104. d	141. a
31. c	68. b	105. d	142. d
32. b	69. c	106. c	143. a
33. d	70. d	107. d	144. a
34. d	71. b	108. b	145. c
35. d	72. d	109. c	
36. d	73. b	110. a	
37. b	74. a	111. b	

REFERENCES

1. American Dental Association, Bureau of Chemistry and Council on Dental Therapeutics: Formulation and packaging of aqueous solutions of sodium fluoride for topical application. J.A.D.A., *38*:142, 1949.
2. American Dental Association, Council on Dental Therapeutics: *Accepted Dental Remedies.* 32nd ed. Chicago, American Dental Association, 1967.
3. American National Red Cross: *First Aid Textbook.* 4th Ed. Garden City, Doubleday & Co., Inc., 1957.
4. Angle, E. H.: *Malocclusion of the Teeth.* 7th Ed. Philadelphia, S. S. White, 1907.

5. Baer, P. N., and Newton, W. L.: Occurrence of periodontal disease in germ-free rats. J. Dent. Res., *38*:1238, 1959.
6. Baer, P. N., and Newton, W. L.: Studies on periodontal disease in the mouse. III. The germ-free mouse and its conventional control. Oral Surg., Oral Med. & Oral Path., *13*:1134, 1960.
7. Bhaskar, S. N.: *Synopsis of Oral Pathology*. St. Louis, C. V. Mosby Co., 1961.
8. Bibby, B. G.: Diet and dental health. Nutrition News, *30*:1, 1967.
9. Bibby, B. G.: *Local Effects of Nutrients in Nutrition and Caries Prevention*. Stockholm, Almquist & Wiksell, 1965.
10. Brudevold, F.: Action of topically applied fluoride. J. Dent. Child., *26*:186, 1959.
11. Brudevold, F.: Fluorides in the prevention of dental caries. Dent. Clin. North America, 397, July, 1962.
12. Burket, L. W.: *Oral Medicine*. 4th Ed. Philadelphia, Lippincott, 1961.
13. Carter, C. F., and Smith, A. L.: *Microbiology and Pathology*. St. Louis, C. V. Mosby Co., 1956.
14. Finn, S. B.: *Clinical Pedodontics*. 2nd Ed. Philadelphia, W. B. Saunders Co., 1962.
15. Fitzgerald, R. J., and McDaniel, E. G.: Dental calculus in the germ-free rat. Arch. Oral Biol., *2*:239, 1960.
16. Glickman, I.: *Clinical Periodontology*. 2nd Ed. Philadelphia, W. B. Saunders Co., 1958.
17. Gustafsson, B. E., Quensel, C. E., Lanke, L. S., Lundquist, C., Grahnen, H., Bonow, B. E., and Krasse, B.: The effect of different levels of carbohydrate intake on caries activity in 436 individuals observed for five years. Acta Odont. Scandinav., *16*: 232, 1954.
18. Jay, P.: The reduction of oral lactobacillus acidophilus counts by the periodic restriction of carbohydrate. Amer. J. Orthodont. & Oral Surg., *33*:162, 1947.
19. Jay, P., Beeuwkes, A. M., and MacDonald, H. B.: *Dietary Program for the Control of Dental Caries*. Ann Arbor, the Overbeck Co., 1959.
20. Muhler, J. C.: Anticariogenic effectiveness of a single application of stannous fluoride in children residing in an optimal communal fluoride area. II. Results at the end of 30 months. J.A.D.A., *61*:431, 1960.
21. Pameijer, J. H. N., Brudevold, F., and Hunt, E. E., Jr.: A study of acidulated fluoride solutions. III. The cariostatic effect of repeated topical sodium fluoride applications with and without phosphate. A pilot study. Arch. Oral Biol., *8*:183, 1963.
22. Peterson, S.: *Clinical Dental Hygiene*. 2nd Ed. St. Louis, C. V. Mosby Co., 1963.
23. Sicher, H.: *Orban's Oral Histology and Embryology*. 5th Ed. St. Louis, C. V. Mosby Co., 1962.
24. Steele, P. F.: *Dimensions of Dental Hygiene*. Philadelphia, Lea & Febiger, 1966.
25. Stephan, R. M.: Changes in hydrogen-ion concentrations on tooth surfaces and in carious lesions. J.A.D.A., *27*:718, 1940.
26. Stephan, R. M.: Intra-oral hydrogen-ion concentrations associated with dental caries activity. J. Dent. Res., *23*:257, 1944.
27. Stoll, F. A., and Catherman, J. L.: *Dental Health Education*. 3rd Ed. Philadelphia, Lea & Febiger, 1967.
28. Thoma, K. H., and Goldman, H. M.: *Oral Pathology*. 5th Ed. St. Louis, C. V. Mosby Co., 1960.
29. Weidmann, S. M.: Review of modern concepts on calcification. Arch. Oral Biol., *1*:259, 1960.
30. Wellock, W. D., and Brudevold, F.: A study of acidulated fluoride solutions. II. The caries inhibiting effect of single annual topical applications of an acidic fluoride and phosphate solution. A two year experience. Arch. Oral Biol., *8*:179, 1963.
31. Wellock, W. D., Maitland, A., and Brudevold, F.: Caries increments, tooth discoloration, and state of oral hygiene in children given single annual applications of acid phosphate-fluoride and stannous fluoride. Arch. Oral Biol., *10*:453, 1965.
32. Wilkins, E. M., and McCullough, P. A.: *Clinical Practice of the Dental Hygienist*. 2nd Ed. Philadelphia, Lea & Febiger, 1964.

CHAPTER 10

DENTAL MATERIALS

James Overberger

1. Once a dental product is found to comply with the requirements of the respective American Dental Association Specification, its name is placed on the list of

   a. Certified Dental Materials
   b. Best Dental Materials
   c. Popular Dental Materials
   d. Approved Dental Materials

2. The American Dental Association Specifications contain certain requirements for physical and chemical properties of dental materials which will ensure

   a. their quality and usefulness to the dentist
   b. superior dental restorations
   c. high profits for the manufacturer
   d. low material cost for the dentist

3. Compressive stress is computed by dividing the external force by the

   a. length of the test specimen
   b. area of the test specimen
   c. strain of the test specimen
   d. elasticity of the test specimen

4. Hardness is measured by means of

   a. indentation tests
   b. tensile tests
   c. compression tests
   d. strain tests

5. The process by which atoms and molecules return to their normal positions relieving stress and strain is known as

    a. relaxation
    b. expansion
    c. contraction
    d. diffusion

6. The ability of a material to withstand permanent deformation under tensile stress without fracture is known as

    a. malleability
    b. ductility
    c. hardness
    d. flow

7. The greatest stress that a structure can withstand without rupture is known as the

    a. hardness
    b. yield strength
    c. ultimate strength
    d. ductility

8. Materials that are placed in close proximity to vital pulpal tissues should have

    a. high thermal conductivity
    b. low thermal conductivity
    c. high copper oxide content
    d. high acid content

9. The modulus of elasticity is a measure of the

    a. strength of a material
    b. rigidity or stiffness of a material
    c. ability to be stressed with plastic deformation
    d. ductility or malleability of a material

10. The material that most closely approximates the coefficient of expansion and contraction of tooth structure is

    a. amalgam
    b. casting gold alloy
    c. acrylic resin
    d. silicate cement

11. A crystalline material is distinguished from an amorphous material by its

    a. regular atomic or molecular arrangement
    b. irregular atomic or molecular arrangement
    c. lack of definite melting or freezing point
    d. flow under load

12. Stress induced in a structure as a result of a load application varies

    a. directly with the length
    b. inversely with the melting range
    c. inversely with the load and directly with the cross sectional area
    d. directly with the load and inversely with the cross sectional area

13. The key to the optimum physical and manipulative properties of gypsum products is the use of

    a. vacuum mixing
    b. chemical modifiers
    c. the proper water/powder ratio
    d. a flexible bowl and stiff spatula

14. The chemical formula of the mineral gypsum used as a raw material and that of the hardened gypsum product is

    a. $CaSO_4 \cdot 2\ H_2O$
    b. $(CaSO)_2 \cdot \frac{1}{2}\ H_2O$
    c. $(CaSO)_4 \cdot \frac{1}{2}\ H_2O$
    d. $CaSO \cdot 4\ H_2O$

15. The strength of stone exceeds that of plaster because it contains fewer

    a. powder particles
    b. voids
    c. chemical additives
    d. nuclei of crystallization

16. The safest method for soaking a gypsum cast is to place it in

    a. boiling water for ten minutes
    b. room temperature water overnight
    c. room temperature gypsum slurry water until saturated
    d. running warm tap water for fifteen minutes

17. A better stone surface will be obtained from a reversible hydrocolloid impression if the stone hardens in

    a. water
    b. air
    c. 100% relative humidity
    d. 2% potassium sulfate solution

18. The physical character of the powder particles of dental stone is described as

    a. smooth and porous
    b. smooth and nonporous
    c. rough and nonporous
    d. rough and porous

19. All of the following agents will retard the setting of gypsum products *except*

    a. agar agar
    b. sodium citrate
    c. borax
    d. potassium sulfate

20. The best method for routinely obtaining a cast with optimum surface characteristics is to

    a. soak the cast in molten petrolatum
    b. use correctly manipulated densite stone
    c. use a high water-powder ratio of the selected gypsum product
    d. soak the cast in mineral oil

21. Which of the following dental gypsum products exhibits the greatest setting expansion?

    a. plaster
    b. stone
    c. improved (densite) stone

22. On a hot humid day, the zinc-oxide eugenol impression materials may exhibit a short working time which is due to

    a. the increased exothermic heat of reaction
    b. their sensitivity to heat and humidity
    c. the increased dissociation of the eugenol
    d. the accelerating effect of the zinc acetate

23. The main ingredients of impression compound are a
   a. thermoplastic resin, a plasticizer, and filler
   b. thermosetting resin, a plasticizer, and filler
   c. thermosetting resin, a plasticizer, and water soluble wax
   d. thermoplastic resin, inert filler, and a chemical accelerator

24. The process by which an exudate forms on the surface of an alginate impression is called
   a. syneresis
   b. imbibition
   c. evaporation
   d. osmosis

25. The basic constituent of reversible hydrocolloid impression materials is
   a. agar agar
   b. alginic acid
   c. gelatin
   d. polyvinyl chloride

26. The basic ingredient of irreversible hydrocolloid impression material is
   a. a complex silicofluoride
   b. a soluble alginate
   c. gelatin
   d. alginic acid

27. After initial gelation of regular setting irreversible hydrocolloid impression material, the impression should be removed from the mouth
   a. immediately
   b. after 2 to 3 minutes
   c. slowly
   d. after 5 to 6 minutes

28. An alginate impression should be poured
   a. immediately
   b. after 20 minutes
   c. after 30 minutes
   d. after 40 minutes

29. The usual reactor used for polymerizing polysulfide rubber impression materials is
   a. lead peroxide
   b. tin octoate
   c. silver peroxide
   d. benzoyl peroxide

30. When using rubber impression materials, more accurate results will be obtained when the impression material is

   a. evenly distributed and of minimum thickness
   b. bulky and thick
   c. used in a compound tray
   d. used in a plastic stock tray

31. Which one of the following impression materials is the most dimensionally stable?

   a. impression compound
   b. alginate hydrocolloid
   c. agar hydrocolloid
   d. zinc-oxide eugenol impression paste

32. Moisture contamination of alginate impression material is to be avoided to prevent

   a. stress relaxation of the set material
   b. a chalky appearance forming on the cast surface
   c. tackiness to the surface of the gel
   d. erratic setting times

33. A rubber impression should not be removed from the mouth until sufficient elasticity is developed in the material, generally _____ minutes after the material is carried to the mouth.

   a. 2
   b. 4
   c. 8
   d. 16

34. The sol-gel transformation of agar impression materials is a

   a. chemical reaction
   b. physical reaction
   c. combination of chemical and physical reaction
   d. chelation reaction

35. The best method for the dentist to control the gelation time of irreversible hydrocolloid impression material is to alter the

   a. temperature of the mix water
   b. water-powder ratio
   c. mixing time
   d. composition

36. The reaction between zinc oxide and eugenol is a complex chemical reaction in which

   a. surface reacted particles of zinc oxide are bonded together by a matrix of zinc eugenolate
   b. completely reacted particles of zinc oxide are bonded together by a matrix of eugenol
   c. surface reacted particles of zinc oxide are bonded together by rosin, inert oils, and zinc chelate
   d. thin crystals of zinc eugenolate precipitate from the setting matrix

37. Dental cements retain restorations in place by forming a(an) _____ between the tooth and restoration.

   a. adhesive bond
   b. mechanical interlocking
   c. chemical bond
   d. covalent bond

38. The essential ingredient of the liquid of zinc phosphate and silicate cement is

   a. acetic acid
   b. phosphoric acid
   c. lactic acid
   d. benzoic acid

39. If a silicate cement restoration is exposed to saliva during the initial phase of setting, its _____ will be increased.

   a. strength
   b. translucency
   c. resistance to staining
   d. solubility

40. The mixing technique for silicate cement can be described as a

   a. folding action over a small area of the slab
   b. vigorous spatulating action over a small area of the slab
   c. vigorous spatulating action over a large area of the slab
   d. folding action over a large area of the slab

41. The main ingredient of the powder of zinc phosphate cement is

   a. tertiary zinc phosphate
   b. magnesium oxide
   c. phosphorus oxide
   d. zinc oxide

42. The least irritating of all the cements is

   a. silicate cement
   b. zinc phosphate cement
   c. copper cement
   d. zinc oxide-eugenol cement

43. The fluorine fluxes present in a silicate cement will

   a. reduce the solubility of the cement and adjacent enamel
   b. improve the manipulative properties
   c. have no effect on either the solubility of the cement or enamel
   d. increase the solubility of the adjacent enamel and cement

44. The final reaction product between zinc phosphate cement powder and liquid is best described as

   a. crystalline in structure with the partially dissolved powder particles suspended in crystals of zinc phosphate compounds
   b. gel in structure with the partially dissolved powder particles suspended in a gel framework of zinc phosphate compounds
   c. crystalline in structure with the powder particles completely dissolved in crystals of zinc phosphate compounds
   d. crystalline in structure with the partially dissolved powder particles suspended in crystals of zinc eugenolate

45. The best method for providing sufficient time for manipulation and incorporation of the maximum amount of powder in a given quantity of liquid for the desired consistency of zinc phosphate cement is to

   a. cool the mixing slab
   b. add all the powder in one increment
   c. prolong the mixing time
   d. dilute the powder

46. Changing the properties of a gold casting by exposing it to elevated temperatures for various periods of time before cooling is due to

   a. heat treatment
   b. grain growth
   c. nuclei treatment
   d. hot working

47. The relative number of grains per unit area of a dental casting is important because the greater the number of grains per unit area the greater the

   a. strength
   b. modulus of elasticity
   c. density
   d. thermal conductivity

48. The increase in values of mechanical properties that accompanies cold working is due to

   a. grain growth
   b. strain hardening
   c. annealing
   d. recovery

49. A gold foil restoration can be fabricated in the prepared cavity of the tooth because of the ability of the gold foil to be _____ at mouth temperature.

   a. cast
   b. welded
   c. forged
   d. soldered

50. Wrought gold alloys have a microscopic structure that is described as

   a. equiaxed
   b. fibrous
   c. columnar
   d. stratified

51. An alloy in which the atoms of the constituent metals are randomly distributed throughout the space lattice of the solid alloy is called

   a. a solid solution alloy
   b. an intermediate compound alloy
   c. an eutectic alloy
   d. a cored alloy

52. Base metal contamination of a casting gold alloy will make the casting

   a. harder
   b. more ductile
   c. stronger
   d. more brittle

53. Which of the following is considered a metalloid?

   a. tin
   b. chromium
   c. nickel
   d. silicon

54. The higher the platinum and palladium content of a casting gold alloy, the

   a. stronger and harder the alloy
   b. weaker and softer the alloy
   c. deeper yellow the color of the alloy
   d. lower the melting range of the alloy

55. The principal constituent responsible for hardening heat treatment of casting gold alloys is

   a. zinc
   b. silver
   c. gold
   d. copper

56. If a dental gold casting made from type III alloy is quenched from a cherry-red color, it will be in a

   a. hardened condition
   b. softened condition
   c. recovery condition
   d. eutectic condition

57. Shrink-spot porosity in a dental gold casting is generally caused by

   a. insufficient molten metal during solidification
   b. gas inclusions
   c. investment inclusions
   d. incomplete wax elimination

58. A properly melted casting gold alloy is best described as having a

   a. dull cloudy surface
   b. mirror-like brilliant surface
   c. greenish-yellow dull surface
   d. bluish-silver dull surface

59. A flux may be added to the molten gold alloy before casting in order to

   a. remove any oxides on the surface of the alloy
   b. decrease the melting range of the alloy
   c. keep the asbestos liner from breaking apart
   d. act as a lubricant for entrance of the molten gold into the sprue hole

60. The proper zone of a gas-air blowpipe flame used for melting casting gold alloys is the

    a. reducing zone
    b. oxidizing zone
    c. zone nearest the nozzle
    d. outermost zone

61. A defective casting made in an investment that does not contain a reducing agent that exhibits rounded margins and a shiny appearance would most likely be caused by

    a. incomplete wax elimination
    b. insufficient casting pressure
    c. use of a small diameter sprue pin
    d. use of too much flux

62. Graphite and powdered copper are added to some casting investments to provide for

    a. increased thermal expansion
    b. increased hygroscopic expansion
    c. an oxidizing atmosphere in the mold at casting
    d. a reducing atmosphere in the mold at casting

63. The amount of effective setting expansion of an investment may vary depending upon the

    a. composition of the wax and type of pattern
    b. type of casting machine used
    c. type of sprue pin used
    d. type of gold alloy used

64. The strength of an investment is mainly controlled by the amount of

    a. binder present
    b. silica present
    c. chemicals present
    d. reducing agents present

65. Of the refractories used in casting investment, _____ has the highest thermal expansion.

    a. quartz
    b. cristobalite
    c. silicate
    d. phosphate

66. The process by which the surface of a casting is cleaned by using acids to remove surface oxides and tarnish is called

    a. pickling
    b. etching
    c. stripping
    d. plating

67. The main ingredient of a typical inlay wax is

    a. beeswax
    b. paraffin wax
    c. wool wax
    d. carnauba wax

68. When using the water bath immersion hygroscopic technique, the size of the casting can be theoretically increased by using a

    a. lower water/powder ratio
    b. higher water/powder ratio
    c. delayed time of immersion
    d. chemical additive

69. The major cause of distortion of a wax pattern is due to the

    a. composition of the wax
    b. relaxation of stresses induced during manipulation
    c. method of heating the wax
    d. use of the direct technique

70. Nodules found on a gold casting are caused by

    a. occluding gases during melting
    b. particles of flux on the surface of the molten gold alloy
    c. trapping air bubbles on the pattern during investing
    d. trapping investment particles on the pattern during investing

71. The ingredient responsible for the deleterious effect of moisture contamination in dental amalgam is

    a. silver
    b. copper
    c. tin
    d. zinc

72. Any manipulation of dental amalgam which tends to increase the amount of solution of mercury in the alloy particles and which decreases the formation of the matrix phases will tend to

    a. decrease the subsequent expansion during hardening
    b. decrease the subsequent contraction during hardening
    c. increase the particle size of the alloy particles
    d. increase the response to aging

73. The dental amalgam restoration is not finished until it is polished, because the procedure

    a. reduces surface roughness and provides a surface more resistant to corrosion
    b. increases the surface hardness of the restoration
    c. reduces the solubility of the adjacent enamel
    d. increases the mercury content of the restoration

74. If excessive mercury is used in the original alloy/mercury ratio, a (an) _____ amount of mercury may be left in the restoration.

    a. lower
    b. higher
    c. equal
    d. optimum

75. Mechanical amalgamation can be used instead of hand amalgamation as this method provides for

    a. increased strength of the amalgam
    b. standardization of the procedure and a reduction of time of amalgamation
    c. increased expansion of the amalgam
    d. decreased flow of the amalgam

76. The presence of tin in the amalgam alloy provides for

    a. an increase in strength and hardness
    b. a decrease in strength and hardness
    c. an increase in expansion
    d. cleanliness of the amalgam during mixing

77. Due to the slow development of strength of amalgam, the patient should be cautioned not to bite hard on a newly condensed amalgam restoration for at least

    a. 6 hours
    b. 9 hours
    c. 12 hours
    d. 15 hours

78. Which statement best describes the setting mechanism of dental amalgam?

    a. The silver-tin compound dissolves mercury and two crystalline phases are formed that bind the partially reacted alloy particles together.

    b. The silver-tin compound dissolves mercury and hardening occurs due to osmotic interaction.

    c. The silver-tin compound dissolves tin and three eutectic phases are formed.

    d. The silver-tin compound dissolves copper and the completely reacted particles bind together.

79. The main effect of increased amalgamation on the properties of amalgam are to

    a. increase the strength and decrease the flow and setting expansion

    b. decrease the strength and increase the flow and setting expansion

    c. increase the strength, flow and setting expansion

    d. decrease the strength, flow and setting expansion

80. Probably the best method for measurement of amalgam alloy in establishing the proper alloy–mercury ratio is to use

    a. a Crandall balance

    b. pre-weighed pellets

    c. a volume dispenser

    d. an estimated amount

81. Once a mix of dental amalgam is made, the amalgam should be

    a. allowed to stand for five minutes

    b. condensed immediately into the prepared cavity

    c. allowed to stand for five minutes and re-amalgamated to ensure good matrix formation

    d. wiped with alcohol to sterilize the amalgam

82. Which of the following variables has the most influence on the strength properties of dental amalgam?

    a. original alloy/mercury ratio

    b. method of amalgamation

    c. method of polishing

    d. final mercury content of the amalgam

83. The chemical process by which the final molecules of denture base acrylic resin are formed is called

    a. polymerization
    b. crystallization
    c. solidification
    d. enucleation

84. A typical temperature cycle for processing acrylic resin in a water bath is

    a. 8 hours or longer at 165° F.
    b. 1½ hours at 212° F. followed by 1 hour at 165° F.
    c. 6 hours at 165° F.
    d. 1½ hours at 130° F. followed by 1 hour at 165° F.

85. The powder of a heat activated acrylic resin will contain a(an) _____ which will decompose when heated and start the polymerization reaction.

    a. initiator
    b. stabilizer
    c. plasticizer
    d. inhibitor

86. If a denture made of polymethyl methacrylate resin is taken out of the mouth for any extended period of time, it should be kept in

    a. a moist environment
    b. a dry environment
    c. alcohol
    d. acetone

87. Polymethyl methacrylate is classed as a thermoplastic resin; however, it is most commonly used in dentistry in the

    a. premixed form (gel)
    b. thermoset form
    c. precured blank form
    d. powder-liquid form

88. The proper physical stage of the powder-liquid form of polymethyl methacrylate resin for filling the mold space in denture construction is the

    a. sandy stage
    b. sticky stage
    c. doughy stage
    d. rubbery stage

89. The chemical activator used in autopolymerizing denture base resin is found in the

    a. powder
    b. liquid
    c. water bath
    d. initiator

90. Adjacent polymer chains of polymethyl methacrylate resin can be joined together by adding

    a. a stabilizing agent
    b. a cross-linking agent
    c. an inhibiting agent
    d. an initiating agent

91. The color stability of heat activated denture base resin is _____ that of chemically activated denture base resin.

    a. better than
    b. less than
    c. the same as

92. The retaining of water either by imbibition or surface absorption that occurs with polymethyl methacrylate resin is known as

    a. water sorption
    b. capillarity
    c. vapor pressure
    d. surface tension

93. The basic ingredient of modern paint-on gypsum resin separators is

    a. cellophane
    b. a soluble alginate
    c. a silicone lubricant
    d. an insoluble alginate

94. The use of a chemically activated resin rather than a heat activated resin for a minor repair of a denture has the advantage of

    a. increased color stability
    b. increased strength of the repair
    c. higher surface hardness
    d. not usually requiring flasking

95. Which of the following abrasives is used extensively as a polishing agent for teeth and metallic restorations?

   a. diamond
   b. tin oxide
   c. carborundum
   d. tripoli

96. Rouge that is used for laboratory polishing of dental precious metals is

   a. chromium oxide
   b. aluminum oxide
   c. iron oxide
   d. silicon dioxide

97. Any effective polishing technique should be preceded by the use of a coarser abrasive in order to

   a. remove visible scratches before polishing is attempted
   b. establish visible scratches in which the polishing agent can lodge
   c. establish scratches for cooling during polishing
   d. ensure the formation of a crystalline surface layer

98. A dental restoration should be highly polished as this will

   a. aid in preventing flow of the restoration
   b. ensure the formation of an abrasive surface on the restoration
   c. aid in preventing tarnish and corrosion
   d. increase the surface hardness of the restoration

99. The hardest and most effective abrasive for tooth enamel is

   a. carbide
   b. diamond
   c. garnet
   d. emery

100. In order for an abrasive to be effective, it should

   a. be harder than the surface to be abraded
   b. have a smooth, brittle edge
   c. be loosely attached to the binder
   d. be strain hardened during cutting

ANSWERS

1. a	26. b	51. a	76. b
2. a	27. b	52. d	77. a
3. b	28. a	53. d	78. a
4. a	29. a	54. a	79. a
5. a	30. a	55. d	80. b
6. b	31. d	56. b	81. b
7. c	32. d	57. a	82. d
8. b	33. c	58. b	83. a
9. b	34. b	59. a	84. a
10. d	35. a	60. a	85. a
11. a	36. a	61. a	86. a
12. d	37. b	62. d	87. d
13. c	38. b	63. a	88. c
14. a	39. d	64. a	89. b
15. b	40. a	65. b	90. b
16. c	41. d	66. a	91. a
17. c	42. d	67. b	92. a
18. b	43. a	68. a	93. b
19. d	44. a	69. b	94. d
20. b	45. a	70. c	95. b
21. a	46. a	71. d	96. c
22. b	47. a	72. a	97. a
23. a	48. b	73. a	98. c
24. a	49. b	74. b	99. b
25. a	50. b	75. b	100. a

REFERENCES

1. Peyton, F. A. et al.: *Restorative Dental Materials.* 2nd Ed., St. Louis, C. V. Mosby Co., 1964.
2. Phillips, R. W., and Skinner, E. W.: *Elements of Dental Materials.* Philadelphia, W. B. Saunders Co., 1965.
3. Taylor, D. F.: Dental Assisting, Course IV, Dental Materials and Technical Procedures. University of North Carolina, School of Dentistry, Chapel Hill. 1965.

CHAPTER 11

ORAL ANATOMY

Harold H. Boyers

1. The form of the deciduous maxillary cuspid differs in several ways from the form of the permanent tooth which replaces it. An important distinguishing feature is

    a. the distal ridge of the cusp is shorter than the mesial ridge
    b. the mesial ridge of the cusp is shorter than the distal ridge
    c. the apex of the root may be inclined toward the lingual
    d. in the labial aspect, the tip of the cusp is mesial to the long axis of the root

2. Which one of the following features is present in the permanent maxillary cuspid, but not in the permanent mandibular cuspid?

    a. There is very little bulging of the contact areas.
    b. The mesial ridge of the cusp is shorter than the distal ridge.
    c. The tip of the cusp is labial to the long axis of the root.
    d. The tip of the cusp is lingual to the long axis of the root.

3. When the alignment and occlusion of the posterior permanent teeth are normal, certain areas of opposing teeth will make contact with each other in centric occlusal relation. Which one of the following statements is correct?

    a. The mesiobuccal cusp of the mandibular first molar contacts the occlusal embrasure between the maxillary second bicuspid and first molar.
    b. The tip of the mandibular cuspid occludes lingual to the distal half of the maxillary cuspid.
    c. The mesiobuccal cusp of the maxillary first molar occludes with the buccal groove of the mandibular second molar.
    d. The maxillary third molar occludes with the mandibular second and third molars.

4. As a result of the normal aging process attrition occurs in certain areas of the teeth. The result of attrition of the contact areas will be

    a. a reduction of the vertical dimension
    b. facets on the tips of cusps
    c. a slight reduction in the size of adjacent embrasures
    d. pain in the temporomandibular joint area

5. The terminal movement of the mandible as the teeth are closed into centric occlusion is determined by the

    a. cusp-fossa relationship of opposing teeth
    b. shape of the articular eminence of the temporomandibular joint
    c. strength of the muscles of mastication
    d. ligaments which go from the skull to the mandible

6. An oblique ridge is found

    a. only on a maxillary molar
    b. on a mandibular first bicuspid
    c. on either a maxillary or mandibular molar
    d. on the lingual of an anterior tooth

7. A transverse ridge is most likely to be found on

    a. a deciduous maxillary molar crown
    b. a mandibular first bicuspid
    c. the lingual of a maxillary cuspid crown
    d. the occlusal surface of a maxillary first bicuspid

8. A sulcus is

    a. a deep pit-shaped depression in the surface of the crown of a tooth
    b. a linear depression in the surface of a tooth, the inclines of which meet at an angle
    c. the same as a developmental groove because it marks the junction of lobes
    d. a triangular depression in the enamel surface of a tooth

9. The term "permanent anterior teeth" is applied to

    a. the maxillary incisors only
    b. the maxillary central and lateral incisors and cuspids
    c. the maxillary and mandibular teeth which are mesial to the first bicuspids
    d. the maxillary and mandibular central and lateral incisors

10. The term abrasion, as used in dentistry, refers to the

   a. normal wearing away of tooth substances due only to the effects of mastication
   b. wearing away of tooth substances due to the stresses of mastication and/or mechanical means
   c. wearing away of tooth substance at only areas which are in contact with adjacent teeth
   d. removal of tooth substance during the process of preparing a tooth for a restoration

11. Select the proper arrangement of letters to indicate the usual order of eruption of the deciduous teeth. The letters shall designate the teeth as follows: A—central, B—lateral, C—cuspid,—D—first molar, and E—second molar.

   a. A B C D E
   b. A B D E C
   c. A B D C E

12. Calcification of the permanent first molar starts

   a. two months before birth
   b. at birth or soon thereafter
   c. at the age of one year or soon thereafter

13. Calcification of the deciduous teeth first begins

   a. between the fourteenth and seventeenth week in utero
   b. at the twenty-eighth week in utero
   c. at birth or soon thereafter

14. How many centers of calcification are involved in the formation of the deciduous central incisors?

   a. four
   b. one
   c. three

15. The apical portion of the root of the deciduous maxillary central incisor is fully formed

   a. about one year after the tooth has erupted
   b. about the time the tooth erupts
   c. about 6 months before the tooth erupts

16. The apical portions of the roots of a deciduous maxillary first molar are fully formed

    a. about the time the tooth erupts
    b. about 1½ years after the tooth erupts
    c. about 3 years after the tooth erupts

17. The apical portion of the root of a deciduous maxillary central incisor starts to resorb when a child is about

    a. 3 years old
    b. 4½ years old
    c. 6 years old

18. Many changes must take place in the jaws as the teeth develop and erupt. Which of the following is the most important?

    a. an increase in blood supply to the bones of the jaws
    b. an increase in the vertical dimension of the alveolar processes
    c. the apposition of bone on the inferior portion of the body of the mandible
    d. the development of the gingival mucosa

19. As a child's mandible develops between the ages of one and twelve years, the

    a. angle between the body and ramus becomes more obtuse
    b. angle between the body and ramus becomes less obtuse
    c. apices of the roots of the mandibular third molars are fully formed

20. Several things normally occur in a tooth after it has erupted. Which of the following is the *most* important as far as the health of the tooth is concerned?

    a. The enamel surface becomes stained if a person smokes.
    b. The ameloblasts continue to function.
    c. The odontoblasts continue to function.

21. The maxillary division of the trigeminal nerve passes through the

    a. foramen ovale
    b. foramen rotundum
    c. foramen magnum

22. The nerve which innervates most of the hard palate is the

    a. anterior palatine
    b. middle palatine
    c. posterior palatine

23. The suture between the parietal bones is called the

   a. squamous suture
   b. lamboidal suture
   c. sagittal suture

24. The area in which the frontal, parietal, sphenoid, and temporal bones come together is called the

   a. pterion
   b. nasion
   c. anterior fontanel

25. The strongest of the following muscles is the

   a. masseter
   b. lateral pterygoid
   c. buccinator

26. What movement does the genioglossus muscle cause?

   a. lateral flattening of the tongue
   b. protrusion of the tongue
   c. retraction of the tongue

27. The facial artery is a branch of the

   a. internal carotid artery
   b. external carotid artery
   c. maxillary artery

28. The inferior alveolar artery is a branch of the

   a. maxillary artery
   b. facial artery
   c. posterior superior alveolar artery

29. The group of lymph nodes that is commonly called the "dental group" of lymph nodes is the

   a. submental group
   b. parotid group
   c. submandibular group

30. A knowledge of the lymphatic system of the head is helpful to a dental hygienist because

   a. lymph is a clear viscous liquid
   b. symptoms of certain diseases are first detected in lymph nodes near the diseased area
   c. lymph carries certain nutrients to the individual tissue cells

31. The temporomandibular joint may be adversely affected by certain circumstances, even though an individual has a full complement of teeth which are in normal occlusion. One such condition is

    a. subluxation
    b. strain on the articular disk if the person can exert a great force with his muscles of mastication
    c. arthritis

32. The temporomandibular joint

    a. is unique because it allows a wide range of movements of its component parts
    b. has a capsule which is composed of nonelastic fibers
    c. has an articular disk which is well fixed and stationary

33. The temporomandibular joint, the muscles of mastication, and the ligaments that are closely associated thereto will permit a wide range of movements of the mandible. As a person masticates,

    a. the principal movement is directed vertically
    b. the principal movement is directed laterally
    c. a combination of vertical and lateral movements is involved

34. The body of the tongue is primarily composed of several muscles which are called intrinsic muscles of the tongue. Which of the following statements is true?

    a. The muscle whose fibers run anteroposteriorly causes a flattening of the papillae.
    b. One of these muscles has fibers which are directed transversely or from side to side in the tongue.
    c. If these intrinsic muscles are exceptionally strong, we speak of the person as being tongue-tied.

35. Many small glands are associated with the mucosa of the oral cavity, and the secretions

    a. function to assist in the digestion of food
    b. function to assist in the lubrication of the mucosa
    c. of all these glands are thick and viscous

36. The parotid gland is one of the larger glands associated with the oral cavity which

    a. produces a serous type secretion
    b. empties secretions into Wharton's duct
    c. is innervated by the infraorbital nerve

37. The submandibular salivary gland

    a. was formerly called the submaxillary salivary gland
    b. is the same as the submental salivary gland
    c. is located near the symphysis of the mandible

38. The maxillary sinus

    a. is not closely related to the field of operation of a dental hygien-
       ist, but it is closely related to that of an oral surgeon
    b. is one of the smaller air sinuses of the skull
    c. has an orifice into the nasal cavity in the area inferior to the
       inferior concha

39. There are many tooth form abnormalities which are mostly confined
to the

    a. deciduous dentition
    b. permanent dentition
    c. mandibular teeth
    d. maxillary teeth

40. Supplemental teeth are usually found in the

    a. mandibular incisor area
    b. maxillary incisor area
    c. bicuspid area
    d. molar area

41. A common abnormality of tooth form is

    a. a peg-shaped permanent maxillary lateral
    b. a peg-shaped deciduous maxillary lateral
    c. a permanent maxillary central with a tubercle-shaped cingulum
    d. a deciduous maxillary central with a tubercle-shaped cingulum

42. A cleft lip usually appears

    a. in the midline of the upper lip
    b. lateral to the midline in the upper lip
    c. lateral to the midline in the lower lip
    d. in the midline of the lower lip

43. An abnormality of the labial frenum of the upper lip

    a. is often associated with a diastema
    b. causes the lip to be practically immobile
    c. should be surgically altered in infancy

44. Alveolus means the

    a. bony process of the maxilla or mandible which supports the teeth
    b. so-called socket of a tooth
    c. portion of bone which is adjacent to the lingual surfaces of the roots of the teeth
    d. bone which forms the inferior part of the mandible

45. The geometric form of the occlusal aspect of a five-cusped deciduous mandibular second molar or permanent mandibular first molar is a

    a. square
    b. rhomboid
    c. hexagon
    d. rectangle

46. The pulp tissue of a tooth may show response in several ways to external stimuli. Which of the following are examples?

    A. sensation of heat
    B. sensation of cold
    C. sensation of pain
    D. formation of secondary dentin

    a. A, C, and D
    b. C and D
    c. A, B, C, and D
    d. A, B, and D

47. When the occlusion and alignment of teeth are normal we will find that facets due to attrition will develop in certain areas of the teeth. Which of the following are examples?

    A. labioincisal area of a maxillary lateral incisor
    B. linguoincisal area of a maxillary central incisor
    C. labial side of the cusp of a mandibular cuspid
    D. lingual side of the cusp of a maxillary cuspid

    a. A, C, and D
    b. B, C, and D
    c. A, B, and D
    d. C and D

48. The various types of living tissues respond in specialized ways to stimuli. Which of the following statements illustrate this?

    A. The ligaments of the periodontal membrane are so oriented that they can withstand great stresses which are directed at a right angle to the long axis of a tooth.
    B. The odontoblasts form "secondary" dentin if they are subjected to certain mild stimuli.
    C. The nerve tissue within a tooth will respond to every type of severe stimulation by giving a sensation of pain.
    D. The ameloblasts can be stimulated, after a tooth has erupted, to repair hypoplastic enamel.

    a. A and C
    b. B and C
    c. C and D
    d. B and D

49. In the geometric concept of tooth form, the

    A. occlusal aspect of the maxillary second bicuspid is rectangular
    B. cross section of the root of a maxillary central incisor is triangular
    C. occlusal aspect of a deciduous maxillary second molar is a rhomboid
    D. proximal surface of an incisor is triangular

    a. B and D
    b. B, C, and D
    c. A, B, and D
    d. all of the above

50. The geometric form of a maxillary third molar, in the occlusal aspect, will generally be either one or the other of two forms.

    A. triangular
    B. rhomboidal
    C. square
    D. trapezoidal

    a. A or C
    b. B or D
    c. A or B
    d. B or C

51. The form of certain teeth makes those teeth well suited for special purposes. Which of the following statements illustrate this?

    A. The incisor crowns are somewhat chisel-shaped so that the teeth can bite-off portions of food.

    B. The occlusal surfaces of molars are made up of a series of ridges and grooves so that the teeth can grind food.

    C. The roots of maxillary molars are divergent so that they will not puncture the maxillary sinus as forces of mastication are exerted on the teeth.

    D. The roots of deciduous molars are divergent for the primary purpose of making the teeth more stable in the jaws.

    a. A and C
    b. C and D
    c. A and B
    d. B and C

52. The cingulum often takes the form of a definite tubercle on a

    A. mandibular central or lateral incisor
    B. mandibular cuspid
    C. maxillary cuspid
    D. maxillary lateral incisor

    a. C and D
    b. A and C
    c. B and D
    d. B and C

53. Because the anatomical form of certain teeth is related to alignment, occlusion, and function, the

    A. incisal ridge of the mandibular lateral incisor is rotated on the root so that the crown of the tooth will conform to the curvature of the arch

    B. root of a maxillary central incisor is triangular in cross section so that there will be no impingement on the contents of the incisive foramen

    C. root of the maxillary central incisor is triangular in cross section to prevent rotation of the tooth in the jaw

    D. roots of the maxillary third molars are often fused during development to make the teeth relatively simple to extract

    a. A and C
    b. A, B, and C
    c. B and D
    d. B and A

54. A cusp of Carabelli may be located on the

   A. mesiolingual surface of a deciduous maxillary second molar
   B. mesiolingual surface of any permanent maxillary molar
   C. mesiolingual surface of the permanent maxillary first molar, but
      not in the second and third molars
   D. mesiolingual surface of any deciduous maxillary molar

   a. A and C
   b. B and D
   c. A and B
   d. B and C

55. The cementoenamel junction

   A. of an anterior tooth has a greater curvature on the distal than
      on the mesial side
   B. of a cuspid is convex toward the incisal on the proximal surfaces
   C. delineates the anatomic crown of a tooth
   D. delineates the clinical crown of a tooth

   a. A and C
   b. A and D
   c. B and C
   d. B and D

56. Moving posteriorly from the maxillary first to the second to the
   third molar we find

   A. an increase in the length of the root trunk
   B. less divergence of roots
   C. a reduction in size of, or a loss of, the distolingual cusp
   D. an increased tendency for fusion of the roots and more distal
      inclination of the roots

   a. A and D
   b. C and D
   c. B and D
   d. all of the above

57. Which of the following statements is true?

> A. A prominent cervical enamel ridge is present on the mesiobuccal surface of a permanent mandibular second molar.
> B. A prominent cervical enamel ridge is present on the mesiobuccal surface of a deciduous maxillary first molar.
> C. There isn't a developmental depression at the cementoenamel junction of a maxillary second bicuspid.
> D. The longitudinal developmental groove in the mesial side of the root of a permanent mandibular lateral incisor is deeper than that in the distal side.

> a. B, C and D
> b. A, B and D
> c. A, B and C
> d. A, C, and D

58. When deciduous teeth are compared with permanent teeth, differences are noted in

> A. color
> B. size
> C. thickness of enamel
> D. hardness of enamel

> a. A and B
> b. A, B, and D
> c. B and D
> d. all of the above

59. Several types of stimulation generally cause the formation of secondary dentin such as

> A. a severe blow on a tooth
> B. certain restorative materials
> C. the presence of slowly progressing caries
> D. repeated thermal changes

> a. A and C
> b. A, B, and D
> c. B and C
> d. B, C, and D

60. As secondary dentin is formed in a tooth
    A. the pulp cavity becomes smaller
    B. the tooth becomes less sensitive to thermal changes
    C. the tooth becomes more sensitive to thermal changes
    D. it causes the enamel to become harder

    a. B and D
    b. A and B
    c. A, C, and D
    d. A, B, and D

61. The pulp tissue of a tooth contains
    A. odontoblasts
    B. cementoblasts
    C. pulpoblasts
    D. nerve tissue

    a. A and C
    b. A, B, and C
    c. A and D
    d. A, C, and D

62. When comparing deciduous molars with permanent molars it should
    be noted that the
    A. faciolingual dimension between the cusps is proportionately
       narrower in the deciduous molar
    B. ratio of root length to crown length is greater in the deciduous
       molars
    C. root trunk is relatively longer in the deciduous molars
    D. cusps, before attrition, are not as sharp in the deciduous molars

    a. A and B
    b. B and C
    c. A only
    d. B and D

63. When a deciduous maxillary central incisor is compared with its
    succedaneous tooth,
    A. the ratio of crown length to root length is greater in the decidu-
       ous tooth
    B. the root, in cross section, of the deciduous tooth is very different
       in shape
    C. no mamelons exist on the deciduous tooth, but they do on the
       succedaneous tooth
    D. the crown of the deciduous tooth bulges more in the cervical area

    a. B only
    b. A, C, and D
    c. A and D
    d. B and D

64. The deciduous teeth should perform certain functions such as

    A. acting as space maintainers for the successional teeth
    B. mastication of food
    C. aiding in phonetics
    D. contributing to the pleasing appearance of the child

    a. A, B, and C
    b. A, B, and D
    c. A, C, and D
    d. all of the above

65. The dentition of man is well suited for his way of life because he

    A. is omnivorous
    B. likes a diet composed of meat and vegetables
    C. is primarily carnivorous
    D. is primarily herbivorous

    a. C only
    b. D only
    c. A only
    d. B and D

66. The occlusion of the deciduous dentition differs from that of the permanent dentition because

    A. there is more horizontal overlap in the deciduous dentition
    B. there is less vertical overlap in the deciduous dentition
    C. there is more definite cusp-fossa relationship of opposing molars in the permanent dentition
    D. the jaws of a child are smaller than those of an adult

    a. A and B
    b. B and C
    c. C and D
    d. B and D

67. The ability to masticate food differs between a child and an adult because

    A. of the difference in size between deciduous and permanent teeth
    B. a child with loose deciduous teeth is uncomfortable if he chews very hard
    C. the enamel of deciduous teeth is thin
    D. the pulp cavities of deciduous teeth are relatively large

    a. A and B
    b. A and D
    c. B and C
    d. B and D

68. Many dentists state that the periodontium is protected by certain features of tooth form and alignment, some of which are
    A. the cervical enamel ridge
    B. a snug contact between adjacent teeth
    C. the presence of marginal ridges and associated triangular fossae of posterior teeth
    D. a pronounced vertical overlap of the anterior teeth

    a. A and D
    b. B and C
    c. B and D
    d. A, B, and C

69. The periodontal membrane is composed, in part, of ligaments. Some of these ligaments
    A. are attached to enamel in the adult
    B. are attached to cementum in the adult
    C. act as a "hammock" to withstand the forces of mastication
    D. are parallel to the long axis of the tooth and extend from the apex to the crest of the alveolar bone

    a. A and C
    b. B and C
    c. B and D
    d. C and D

70. During the development of the alveolar processes,
    A. the tips of the cusps of the bicuspids always retain the same relationship or proximity to the bifurcation of the roots of the deciduous teeth
    B. the vertical dimension of the face becomes greater
    C. the mandibular but not the maxillary arch becomes longer
    D. the width of the arches remains constant

    a. A and C
    b. B and C
    c. B only
    d. B and D

71. The process of root resorption of deciduous teeth requires
    A. about 1½ to 2 years for the centrals
    B. about 3 to 4 years for the molars
    C. about 3 to 4 years for the centrals
    D. about 3 to 4 years for the cuspids

    a. A and D
    b. A, B, and D
    c. B, C, and D
    d. C and D

72. Which of the following statements are true and related to the development of the face and head?

A. Several fontanels are present at the time of birth.
B. Several cranial sutures, which are not tightly closed at birth, help to facilitate the process of birth.
C. The maxillary sinuses are large in a young child.
D. The mandibular succedaneous incisor teeth develop lingual to the roots of the deciduous teeth.

a. A, B, and D
b. B, C, and D
c. A and C
d. all of the above

73. Which of the following statements include changes that take place with aging?

A. The permanent teeth usually become somewhat darker.
B. A relatively great amount of incisal attrition takes place by the time the deciduous incisors are exfoliated.
C. The pulp cavities of permanent teeth become smaller.
D. Root shapes change after their apices have formed. (Do not consider change due to hypercementosis or resorption.)

a. A, B, and C
b. A, B, and D
c. B, C, and D
d. C and D

74. The primary function of the alveolar processes of the two jaws is to

a. increase the vertical dimension of the face
b. afford a solid support for the teeth
c. establish the boundaries of the oral cavity
d. mold and shape the tongue

75. The maxillary sinus and the mandibular canal are in close proximity to the apices of the roots of certain teeth in many people. Therefore these facts should always be kept in mind because of the

a. complications which might arise if we have to remove a root fragment
b. likelihood of these structures being injured as the roots of the deciduous teeth are being resorbed
c. likelihood that these structures will be injured by the roots during heavy mastication
d. likelihood that these structures will become calcified as the apices of the roots are becoming calcified

76. If a single injection of a local anesthetic agent is made in order to anesthetize the mandibular teeth on one side of the mouth, the solution is deposited

    a. into the mental foramen
    b. near the lingula
    c. just buccal to the most posterior molar
    d. just lingual to the most posterior molar

77. Swelling in the submental lymph nodes would be most likely to indicate an infection in the

    a. ear
    b. tonsils
    c. mandibular anterior teeth
    d. nasal cavity

78. This diagram represents the cross sectional shape, in the apical aspect, of the root of the

    a. maxillary right cuspid
    b. maxillary right central incisor
    c. maxillary left central incisor
    d. mandibular right first bicuspid

Mesial   Distal

79. This diagram represents the cross sectional shape, at the cervix, of the

    a. maxillary right lateral incisor
    b. maxillary right first bicuspid
    c. mandibular right cuspid
    d. maxillary left cuspid

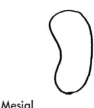

Mesial   Distal

80. This diagram represents the occlusal surface of a permanent mandibular first molar. What is the name of the pattern of grooves?

    a. cross-shape
    b. five-cusp
    c. dryopithecus
    d. pantotherian

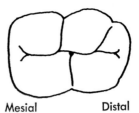

Mesial   Distal

81. This diagram represents the occlusal surface of the

    a. maxillary first bicuspid
    b. maxillary second bicuspid
    c. mandibular first bicuspid
    d. mandibular second bicuspid

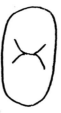

Mesial   Distal

82. This diagram represents the incisal aspect, in geometric form, of the

    a. mandibular right central incisor
    b. mandibular left cuspid
    c. maxillary right lateral incisor
    d. mandibular right lateral incisor

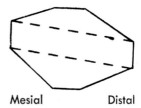

Mesial   Distal

83. This diagram represents the proximal aspect, in geometric form, of the crown of the

    a. maxillary first bicuspid
    b. mandibular second bicuspid
    c. maxillary first molar
    d. mandibular first molar

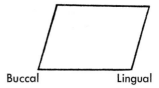

Buccal   Lingual

84. This diagram represents the facial aspect of the

    a. deciduous maxillary left cuspid
    b. deciduous maxillary right cuspid
    c. permanent mandibular left cuspid
    d. deciduous mandibular right cuspid

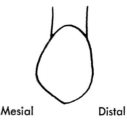

Mesial   Distal

85. This diagram represents the facial aspect for which newly erupted incisor?

    a. permanent maxillary left central
    b. deciduous maxillary left central
    c. permanent maxillary left lateral
    d. deciduous maxillary left lateral

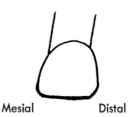

Mesial   Distal

86. A point angle, as used in dentistry, is the

      a. place where several grooves join together
      b. place where several ridges come together
      c. place where three surfaces come together
      d. tip of a cusp

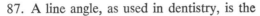

87. A line angle, as used in dentistry, is the

      a. angle between the ramus and body of the mandible
      b. place where two surfaces meet
      c. junction of two lobes or centers of calcification of a tooth
      d. same as an incisal angle

88. The term "col" as used in dentistry

      a. is an abbreviation referring to collection of accounts
      b. is an abbreviation for collar and refers to the cervical line
      c. refers to the shape of the interdental papilla
      d. refers to the shade or color of a tooth

89. The term diastema means a

      a. space between adjacent teeth, usually due to developmental processes
      b. space between adjacent teeth due to a fracture of a tooth
      c. space between adjacent teeth due to loss of a restoration

90. The root resorption process of a deciduous tooth

      a. may start even though a successional tooth is congenitally missing
      b. is not essential to the natural exfoliation of the tooth
      c. is a relatively simple and well understood physiologic process
      d. is initiated by ameloblasts

91. The curve of Spee is

      a. applied only to the bicuspids and molars
      b. applied to anterior and posterior teeth
      c. related to the incisors only
      d. related to the shape of the anterior part of the dental arch

92. Which tooth is most likely to show various crown forms?

      a. deciduous maxillary second molar
      b. deciduous mandibular second molar
      c. maxillary second bicuspid
      d. mandibular second bicuspid

93. Which tooth is most likely to show various root forms?

    a. deciduous maxillary cuspid
    b. deciduous maxillary second molar
    c. permanent maxillary cuspid
    d. permanent mandibular cuspid

94. The usual site of a paramolar cusp is on the

    a. lingual surface of a molar
    b. buccal surface of a molar
    c. distal surface of a molar
    d. occlusal surface of a molar

95. If supplemental teeth are present, they are most likely to be associated with the

    a. deciduous dentition
    b. permanent anterior teeth
    c. bicuspids
    d. permanent mandibular second molars

96. Calcification of a molar first begins at the

    a. dentinoenamel junction of the various cusps
    b. apex of each of the roots
    c. enamel surface of each of the cusps
    d. horns of the pulp

97. The root trunk of a multirooted tooth starts to develop

    a. immediately after the cusps have erupted
    b. prior to the eruption of the cusps
    c. at the same time that the apices start to develop
    d. at the same time that the cusps start to develop

98. In considering the ages of eruption for corresponding teeth of boys and girls, it is observed that

    a. boys' teeth erupt at a younger age
    b. boys' teeth erupt at an older age
    c. boys' and girls' teeth erupt at the same age

99. Occasionally a series of small pits arranged in a horizontal line across the labial surface of the crown of a maxillary central incisor would indicate

    a. an improper toothbrushing technique
    b. a disturbance of the ameloblasts as the tooth was being formed
    c. a disturbance of the odontoblasts as the tooth was being formed
    d. an excessive consumption of carbohydrates as the tooth was being formed

100. One common morphologic feature of the permanent maxillary lateral incisor often leads to a need for a dental restoration because there exists a

    a. deep lingual pit
    b. rounded, obtuse disto-incisal angle
    c. short root
    d. thin incisal ridge

ANSWERS

1. a	26. b	51. c	76. b
2. c	27. b	52. a	77. c
3. a	28. a	53. b	78. b
4. c	29. c	54. c	79. b
5. a	30. b	55. c	80. c
6. a	31. c	56. d	81. b
7. b	32. a	57. c	82. d
8. b	33. c	58. d	83. d
9. c	34. b	59. d	84. a
10. b	35. b	60. b	85. b
11. c	36. a	61. c	86. c
12. b	37. a	62. a	87. b
13. a	38. a	63. b	88. c
14. b	39. b	64. d	89. a
15. a	40. c	65. c	90. a
16. b	41. a	66. b	91. a
17. b	42. b	67. a	92. d
18. b	43. a	68. d	93. d
19. b	44. b	69. b	94. b
20. c	45. c	70. c	95. c
21. b	46. b	71. b	96. a
22. a	47. b	72. a	97. b
23. c	48. b	73. a	98. b
24. a	49. d	74. b	99. b
25. a	50. c	75. a	100. a

REFERENCES

1. Francis, C. C.: *Introduction to Human Anatomy*. 4th Ed. St. Louis, C. V. Mosby Co., 1964.
2. King, B. G., and Showers, M. J.: *Human Anatomy and Physiology*. 5th Ed. Philadelphia, W. B. Saunders Co., 1963.
3. Kraus, B. S., and Jordan, R. E.: *The Human Dentition Before Birth*. Philadelphia, Lea & Febiger, 1965.
4. Scott, J. H., and Symons, N. B.: *Introduction to Dental Anatomy*. 4th Ed. Baltimore, Williams and Wilkins Co., 1964.
5. Sicher, H.: *Oral Anatomy*. 3rd Ed. St. Louis, C. V. Mosby Co., 1960.
6. Wheeler, R. C.: *Textbook of Dental Anatomy and Physiology*. 4th Ed. Philadelphia, W. B. Saunders Co., 1965.

CHAPTER 12

ORAL ROENTGENOLOGY

Camillo A. Alberico

1. A particle substance consisting of a central nucleus surrounded by revolving electrons where the nucleus contains positive proton charges and neutron particles is called

    a. a molecule
    b. a neutron
    c. an atom
    d. an ion

2. Dr. Wilhelm Conrad Roentgen was the discoverer of the x-ray, which has taken his name, the "roentgen ray." In what year did Roentgen discover the x-ray?

    a. 1795
    b. 1845
    c. 1895
    d. 1905

3. X-rays and light belong to the same family of electromagnetic radiations and share the following characteristics.

    A. They affect photographic plates in a similar manner.
    B. They are not affected by magnetic fields.
    C. They travel in straight lines and at the same speed.
    D. They cast shadows of objects in the same manner.
    E. They possess the ability to penetrate opaque objects.

    a. A and B
    b. A, B, and C
    c. B, C, and D
    d. B, D, and E
    e. A, B, C, and D

4. The x-ray machine, when in operation, is capable of producing an electrical force or pressure. The term that describes electrical force or pressure produced in an x-ray machine is

   a. milliampere
   b. volt
   c. kilowatt
   d. ohm

5. The standard unit that is used to measure the amount of electric current flowing through a circuit is the

   a. volt
   b. ohm
   c. ampere
   d. electron

6. The parts of an x-ray machine that are essential to production of roentgen rays are the

   A. autotransformer
   B. step-up transformer
   C. step-down transformer
   D. x-ray tube
   E. milliammeter and timer

   a. A, B, and C
   b. A and D
   c. D and E
   d. A, B, C, and D
   e. all of the above

7. The Coolidge designed roentgen-ray tube eliminated the necessity for gas to create electrons. This tube made it possible to have a heated filament produce electrons. The phenomenon is known as

   A. thermal emission
   B. thermionic emission or incandescence
   C. ionic dispersement
   D. atom cloud formation
   E. electronic scatter

   a. A
   b. B
   c. A and B
   d. C and D
   e. B and E

8. The metallic filament used in the Coolidge or hot filament tube is a special metal called

   a. molybdenum
   b. lead
   c. tungsten
   d. copper

9. A device used in an x-ray machine consisting of two coils of electric wire insulated from each other where the magnetic field around one coil induces an electrical current in the second coil is called

   a. a transformer
   b. a rheostat
   c. an ohm regulator
   d. a resistor

10. A transformer with a single winding, making one coil do the work of two and used for only making minor changes in voltage is known as

    a. a pole transformer
    b. a filament transformer
    c. an autotransformer
    d. an anode transformer

11. Although there are many important factors to be considered when operating x-ray equipment, prime factors necessary for the proper exposure of an x-ray film are

    a. distance and exposure time
    b. milliamperage and kilovoltage
    c. distance and kilovoltage
    d. all of the above

12. An x-ray tube consists of an anode and a cathode enclosed in a highly evacuated glass tube. The tube is supplied with two electrical circuits called

    a. an anode and alternating circuits
    b. a cathode circuit and automatic circuits
    c. anode-cathode and filament circuits
    d. filament and low voltage circuit

13. Electrons are formed at the hot filament of the x-ray tube. When activated these electrons form rays or a stream of electrons that are directed to the target of the x-ray tube, these rays or stream of electrons are called

    a. cathode rays
    b. anode rays
    c. roentgen rays
    d. rays of Geissler

14. The production of x-rays takes place in a tube very similar in appearance to a radio tube. All of the following are necessary for the production of x-rays *except*

    a. production of electrons
    b. a generating system to impart velocity to the electrons
    c. inherent gases to propel the electrons
    d. a target for the sudden stopping of the electrons

15. The manufacturer of an x-ray tube must be very selective of a target material, which ideally possesses

    a. a low atomic number
    b. high vapor pressures at low temperatures
    c. a high melting point
    d. a low degree of thermal conductivity

16. A fundamental difference between the gamma rays of radium and x-rays as indicated by the electromagnetic spectrum is

    a. production of rays
    b. wavelength
    c. rectification
    d. x-rays can be focused but gamma rays cannot

17. The unit of measurement used in the upper ranges of the electromagnetic spectrum is the Angstrom unit. The wavelength used in dentistry measures approximately

    a. 10 to 60 A.U.
    b. 0.1 to 6.0 A.U.
    c. 1.0 to 0.6 A.U.
    d. 100 to 600 A.U.

18. Radiation that is direct from the focal spot of the x-ray tube is called

    a. primary radiation
    b. scattered radiation
    c. the electron beam
    d. stray radiation

19. Radiation incident to the useful beam that produces a certain amount of fog on the roentgenogram and reduces detail is called the

    a. primary radiation
    b. filtered radiation
    c. soft radiation
    d. secondary radiation

20. In dentistry, x-radiation is usually restricted to a specific area. The amount of x-ray reaching the patient's face may be controlled by using

    a. an aluminum filter
    b. the x-ray tube window
    c. a lead diaphragm
    d. a tungsten target

21. In intraoral roentgenography the x-ray beam is collimated to allow only a specific area of the patient's face to be exposed. The recommended beam has a diameter of

    a. 3.5 inches at the patient's skin
    b. 2.0 inches at the patient's skin
    c. 1.25 inches at the patient's skin
    d. 2.75 inches at the patient's skin

22. There are effective ways in dentistry to reduce the dose of radiation the patient receives. These include

    A. use of fast films
    B. collimating the beam
    C. higher kilovoltage and milliamperage
    D. increasing the filtration

    a. A
    b. A and C
    c. B, C, and D
    d. A, B, and D
    e. all of the above

23. By raising the temperature of the cathode filament, a change takes place in the x-ray tube, which

    a. increases the tube milliamperage
    b. increases both milliamperage and kilovoltage
    c. decreases kilovoltage
    d. causes none of the above

24. The area on the target of the anode which is bombarded by the electron stream when the x-ray tube is activated is called the

    a. filament
    b. focal spot
    c. radiator
    d. conductor

25. The most important physical factor in obtaining good image sharpness on a roentgenogram is the

    a. size of the collimator
    b. size of the focal spot area
    c. angle of the tungsten target
    d. proper fixation

26. When referring to the fine delineation of the very small structural elements of the objects in the roentgenogram, reference is being made to

    a. density
    b. contrast
    c. detail
    d. penetration

27. The distance between the focal spot of the x-ray tube and the film affects

    a. detail
    b. penetration
    c. density
    d. contrast

28. Physical factors that must be considered when an exposed film presents geometric unsharpness are

    A. object-film distance
    B. grain size
    C. size of focal area
    D. milliamperage
    E. target-film distance

    a. A, B, and C
    b. A, B, and D
    c. B, C, and D
    d. B, C, and E
    e. A, C, and E

29. Physical factors in film quality that must be considered in regard to density are

    A. kilovoltage peak
    B. fog
    C. milliamperage per unit time
    D. grain size of the film
    E. background scatter

    a. A, B, and C
    b. A, C, and E
    c. B, C, and D
    d. B, D, and E
    e. A, B, and E

30. It is possible to minimize enlargement of the exposed structures farthest from the film by

    A. increasing the target-object distance as far as practical
    B. increasing the size of the focal spot
    C. decreasing the object-film distance
    D. decreasing the target-object distance
    E. decreasing the diaphragm size

    a. A and B
    b. A and C
    c. A, B, and C
    d. B and D
    e. C, D, and E

31. When the low kilovolt range of the x-ray machine is being used, an increase of 10 kilovolts

    a. will not affect the film density
    b. will cause a minimum amount of change in density
    c. will double the density
    d. tends to decrease the overall density

32. The maximum permissible dose of radiation to the operator of an x-ray machine is

    a. three roentgens per year
    b. five roentgens per year
    c. seventy-five roentgens per year
    d. three hundred milliroentgens per week

33. The most important single factor in protecting the patient from excessive radiation is the

    a. speed of the film
    b. proper filtration
    c. exact collimation
    d. cone distance

34. During which period of gestation should the greatest precaution be taken in irradiating the patient?

    a. first trimester
    b. second trimester
    c. third trimester
    d. last two weeks of pregnancy

35. The density of a roentgenogram is *not* affected by

    a. milliamperes per unit time
    b. kilovoltage peak
    c. focal-spot area
    d. fog

36. A dental film upon being exposed and processed will demonstrate, unless protected, a fog due to other than primary radiation. The film is protected by the

   a. outer wrapping paper
   b. black interwrap
   c. lead foil
   d. ultrafast emulsion

37. When the body is exposed to radiation, the amount absorbed is regulated by the

   A. total amount of radiation reaching the area
   B. structure of the part
   C. thickness of the part
   D. quality of radiation

   a. A and D
   b. B and C
   c. A, B, and C
   d. all of the above

38. The x-ray film is made up of a base material coated with an emulsion on either one or both sides. This emulsion is composed of minute particles of

   a. silver nitrate
   b. black metallic silver suspended in gelatin
   c. silver bromide suspended in gelatin
   d. silver nitrate and gelatin
   e. potassium bromide

39. In the developing solution, there are chemicals that have a definite action on a photographic emulsion. The chemicals that definitely liberate the metals from their salts are

   A. hydroquinone
   B. metol or elon
   C. acetic acid
   D. sodium carbonate
   E. sodium thiosulphate

   a. A and C
   b. B and D
   c. A and B
   d. B, C, and D
   e. all of the above

40. A preserving agent must be utilized in developing solutions, otherwise the developing agents would rapidly be exhausted by oxidation. The preserving agent is

    a. potassium bromide
    b. sodium carbonate
    c. hydroquinone
    d. sodium sulfite

41. A "clearing agent" used in the x-ray fixing solution is

    a. ammonium thiosulfate
    b. sodium sulfite
    c. sulfuric acid
    d. aluminum chloride

42. In order to obtain the most consistent results in processing films, the method most accepted is

    a. the visual method
    b. the factoral method
    c. the time-temperature method
    d. a combination of visual-factoral methods

43. The function of a developing solution is to

    A. blacken those parts of the emulsion that have been exposed
    B. clear the film
    C. produce various shades of gray when the film has only been partially exposed
    D. hold down the swelling of the emulsion
    E. not affect those parts of the film that have received no exposure

    a. A
    b. A, B, and C
    c. A, C, and D
    d. A, C, and E
    e. all of the above

44. The sensitive emulsion of the roentgenographic film is changed when the x-ray beam strikes it. This change establishes the

    a. light color changes
    b. dark color changes
    c. latent image
    d. clear areas

45. The penetrating power of an x-ray beam is determined by its effective wavelength. The most effective wavelength would be

   a. the long wavelength
   b. the short wavelength
   c. that created by a low kilovoltage peak
   d. that created by high milliamperage

46. A low contrast image may be produced by using a

   a. high kilovolt beam
   b. low kilovolt beam
   c. short cone
   d. long cone

47. The distortion brought about by a short focal-film distance or by a great object-film distance is called

   a. preshortening
   b. elongation
   c. magnification
   d. cone alteration

48. Shape or true distortion is a result of improper

   A. alignment of the film
   B. focal-film distance
   C. object-film distance
   D. alignment of the useful beam
   E. alignment of the object

   a. A
   b. B and C
   c. A, B, and C
   d. A, C, and E
   e. all of the above

49. One of the physical factors for obtaining optimum definition on a roentgenogram is focal spot size, which is governed by the

   A. filament shape
   B. type of metal used
   C. positioning of the filament in the focusing cup
   D. angle formed by the target surface
   E. distance between the anode and cathode

   a. A and B
   b. B, C, and D
   c. A, B, and C
   d. B, D, and E
   e. A, C, D, and E

50. A roentgenogram may not demonstrate the full length of an object, that is, a foreshortened object, because

    a. the vertical angulation is too great
    b. there is not enough vertical angulation
    c. the horizontal angle is improperly placed
    d. none of the above

51. A processed film that presents a yellowish-brown stain may be the result of

    A. old film
    B. unsafe safelight
    C. light leaking into the darkroom
    D. failure to rinse film before fixer transfer
    E. high-temperature development and a weak fixer

    a. A, B, and C
    b. B and C
    c. D and E
    d. A, B, and C
    e. A, B, and E

52. When using the bisecting the angle technique, with predetermined angles, it is necessary to observe which of the following factors to produce an acceptable roentgenogram?

    A. The occlusal plane of the teeth should be parallel with the floor.
    B. The mid-sagittal plane of the patient should be perpendicular to the floor.
    C. The horizontal angle of the tube must be properly placed.
    D. The vertical angle of the tube must be properly placed.

    a. A and B
    b. C and D
    c. A, B, and D
    d. all of the above

53. When using the bisection of the angle technique, vertical angulation is governed by

    a. the occlusal plane being parallel to the floor
    b. the ala-tragus line
    c. Cieszynski's "rule of isometry"
    d. the sagittal plane being perpendicular to the floor

54. To all users of ionizing radiation, the term "latent period," should be understood. This latent period is

   a. the period of time between the beginning of an x-ray exposure and the end of the exposure
   b. the period of time interposed between exposure and clinical symptoms of x-radiation
   c. the period of time that elapses between pushing the timer button and waiting for the high voltage transformer to become activated
   d. the period of time required for the shadow image to appear on the processed film

55. The use of old films, stray radiation, or an unsafe darkroom light would most likely cause a

   a. blurred film
   b. very light film
   c. very dark film
   d. fogged film

56. Poor processing results occur when solutions are not properly managed. If a developing solution is old, contaminated, or poorly mixed, the result will be a

   a. dark film
   b. fogged film
   c. very light film
   d. normal film if allowed to remain in the developer

57. Whenever the temperature of the processing solutions is too warm and the time is normal for room temperature, the processed film will be a

   a. light film
   b. fogged film
   c. dark film
   d. clear film

58. Films are often inadvertently developed with a high density. These roentgenograms may be lightened by

   a. the use of an oxidizing solution
   b. replacement into fixing solution
   c. washing the film for a long period of time
   d. the use of a cutting reducing solution

59. Radiation affects all vital tissue depending on dose, area, and sensitivity of the particular tissue. Cells exhibiting the greatest sensitivity to radiation are

   a. lymphocytes
   b. muscle cells
   c. bone cells
   d. brain cells

60. One of the earliest signs of overexposure to x-rays may be

   a. keratoses
   b. erythema
   c. blanching of the tissues
   d. alopecia

61. An instrument used on the x-ray machine that indicates the amount of current passing through the x-ray tube is called the

   a. step-up transformer
   b. kilovoltage regulator
   c. milliammeter
   d. step-down transformer

62. Upon viewing an exposed and processed film, a dark area is observed. The word that would describe the area is

   a. roentgenopaque
   b. roentgenolucent
   c. underexposed
   d. underdeveloped

63. A definite advantage found when using the paralleling principle in oral roentgenology is it lessens

   a. exposure time to the patient
   b. object-film distance
   c. angulation distortion
   d. radiation exposure to the operator

64. To decrease magnification when using the long cone paralleling technique in intraoral roentgenography, the

   a. object-film distance is increased
   b. beam is collimated to a smaller diameter
   c. focal-spot-object distance is increased
   d. target-film distance is decreased

65. A complete series of roentgenograms usually contains both periapical and bite-wing films. The bite-wing roentgenogram is especially important to the x-ray examination for identifying

    a. pulp exposures
    b. the proper depth of occlusal caries
    c. proximal carious lesions
    d. the depth of pocket formation

66. When examining a roentgenogram of the maxillary first molar the buccal roots are found to be considerably foreshortened, as a result of

    a. mesially-directed horizontal angulation
    b. too great vertical angulation
    c. too little vertical angulation
    d. none of the above

67. The inverse square law states that the intensity of the useful beam varies inversely as the square of the distance. When using an ultra-fast film with an eight-inch cone and an exposure time of $\frac{5}{10}$ of a second; the exposure time using a sixteen-inch long cone and ultra fast film will be

    a. one second
    b. two seconds
    c. four seconds
    d. three-tenths of a second

68. Frequently on roentgenograms of maxillary molars the malar shadow is superimposed upon the roots or crowns of these teeth. This is most likely to occur when the

    a. long-cone paralleling technique is used
    b. LeMaster's technique is used
    c. bisection of the angle technique is used
    d. short-cone paralleling technique is used

69. Which of the following projections would best locate the position of an impacted mandibular third molar?

    a. a lateral jaw projection
    b. an occlusal projection with a periapical projection
    c. an anterior-posterior projection of the head
    d. a lateral head projection
    e. a Waters projection

70. It is necessary on occasion that extra-oral roentgenograms be exposed in a dental office. A means of lessening radiation to the patient is by using a

    a. film brightener
    b. cardboard film holder
    c. screen film packet
    d. cassette with intensifying screens

71. Occasionally the temperatures of the solutions in a developing tank will vary to such a degree that a processed film, when going from warm to cold, will demonstrate a formation of fine lines in an irregular pattern with a grainy, leather-like appearance. This is referred to as

    a. liquefaction
    b. blistering
    c. reticulation
    d. dichroic fog

72. The screen material used in a cassette fluoresces when struck by x-rays and emits a blue light to which the screen film is very sensitive. The fluorescing material is

    a. calcium tungstate
    b. silver nitrate
    c. silver bromide
    d. calcium carbonate

73. Nonscreen extra-oral film possesses a double emulsion of a thickness greater than that of intra-oral film. The increased emulsion thickness makes this film fast to exposure time; however, because of the increased emulsion the processing time

    a. must be decreased 50% more than other films
    b. must be increased 50% more than other films
    c. must be doubled
    d. will not change because the processing solutions react the same with all types of films

74. One method of localization of an object is to use stereoroentgenography, a method that is valuable because it

    a. allows the viewer to observe from two films
    b. is a simple method of localization
    c. adds perspective or depth to the roentgenogram
    d. necessitates the use of large extra-oral film

75. An intra-oral film that is reversed in film placement will upon being processed present

    a. good density and good definition
    b. good density and poor definition
    c. poor density and poor definition
    d. a very dark film

76. The bisecting technique satisfies which of the following basic principles of shadow casting?

    A. The source of radiation should be as small as possible.
    B. The distance from the light source to the object should be as long as possible.
    C. The distance from the object to the recording surface should be as short as possible.
    D. The object and the recording surface should be parallel.
    E. The light source should strike both the object and recording surface at right angles.

    a. A and C
    b. B and C
    c. A, C, and D
    d. D and E
    e. A, C, D, and E

77. Some objects absorb or offer resistance to the passage of x-radiation. The objects that are not freely penetrable cast a shadow image that is

    a. a dark image
    b. roentgenolucent
    c. roentgenopaque
    d. none of the above

78. Which of the following normal anatomic landmarks appear roentgenolucent on the oral roentgenogram?

    A. mandibular canal
    B. incisive foramen
    C. hamular process
    D. coronoid process
    E. mental foramen

    a. A and B
    b. B and E
    c. C and D
    d. A, B, and C
    e. A, B, and E

79. Which of the following normal anatomic landmarks could be located on a roentgenogram of the maxillary incisor area using the bisecting technique?

    A. tuberosity
    B. incisive foramen
    C. maxillary sinus
    D. nasal septum
    E. median palatine suture line

    a. A and C
    b. B and D
    c. A, C, and E
    d. B, D, and E
    e. A, C, D, and E

80. Which of the following normal anatomic landmarks appear roentgen-opaque on the oral roentgenogram?

    A. maxillary sinus
    B. nasal septum
    C. coronoid process
    D. incisive foramen
    E. hamular process

    a. A, C, and E
    b. B and C
    c. A and D
    d. B, C, and E
    e. A, C, and E

81. Which of the following normal anatomic landmarks could be located on intra-oral roentgenograms of the mandible?

    A. incisive foramen
    B. mental foramen
    C. lingual foramen
    D. external oblique ridge
    E. mylohyoid ridge

    a. A and B
    b. A, C, and E
    c. B and D
    d. B, C, D, and E
    e. all of the above

82. The clear area above the lower anterior incisors is a result of

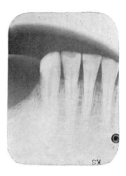

   a. improper developing
   b. improper fixation
   c. improper irradiation with cone-cut
   d. insufficient exposure time

83. When viewing a roentgenogram that is very light and presents several pointed lines, the so-called herringbone effect, one would suspect

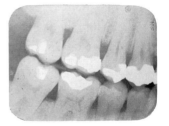

   a. poor processing technique
   b. a film that had been reversed when exposed
   c. a film not sufficiently exposed
   d. old films

84. The white line that appears near the center of the film between the maxillary central incisor and the maxillary cuspid is the result of

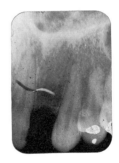

   a. light getting to the film
   b. creasing the film before exposure
   c. the emulsion being scratched from the film base
   d. not blotting saliva from the film packet

85. Excessive density and two images result when a film is

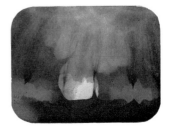

   a. processed a second time
   b. reversed when exposed
   c. processed with double emulsion
   d. inadvertently exposed twice

86. The black line seen in the center of this roentgenogram is caused by

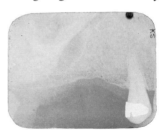

    a. static electricity
    b. scratching the film
    c. improper blotting of the film
    d. placing pressure on the film

87. The roentgenolucent area immediately above the maxillary first molar and bordering the maxillary second bicuspid is the

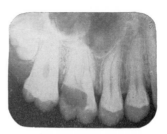

    a. zygoma
    b. maxillary sinus
    c. zygomatic process of the maxilla
    d. nasal fossae

88. The small round roentgenolucent shadow viewed directly below the lower anterior incisors is called the

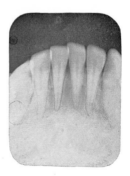

    a. lingual foramen
    b. incisive foramen
    c. genial tubercle
    d. mental protuberance

89. The type of roentgenogram which provides an excellent view of caries, overhanging fillings, and the crest of the ridge is called

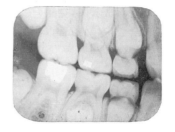

    a. a periapical film
    b. a bite-wing film
    c. an occlusal film
    d. a lateral jaw film

90. The thin roentgenolucent line running between the roots of the central incisors to the crest of the ridge is called the

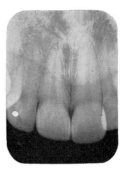

    a. incisive line
    b. median suture line
    c. incisive canal
    d. nasal septum

91. The round normal anatomic roentgenolucent shadow near the apex of the lower left first bicuspid is the

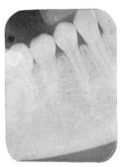

    a. mandibular foramen
    b. mental foramen
    c. lingual foramen
    d. incisive canal

92. The two white roentgenopaque lines lying below the apices of the posterior molar area and above the lower border of the mandible demonstrate normal anatomy. They represent the

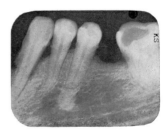

    a. mandibular canal
    b. lingual canal
    c. mental ridges
    d. external oblique ridge

93. The tapered, triangular roentgenopacity at the extreme right of the roentgenogram in the area of the tuberosity and distal to the last molar is a normal anatomic process called the

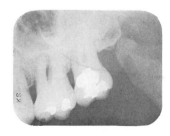

    a. hamular process
    b. zygomatic process
    c. coronoid process
    d. condylar process

94. The roentgenopaque area extending directly above and away from the apices of the central incisors is a normal anatomic landmark called the

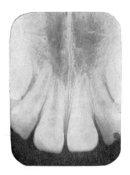

    a. incisive ridge
    b. incisive canal
    c. nasal septum
    d. median palatine suture

95. The roentgenolucent shadows well above the maxillary incisors, bordered and divided by roentgenopaque lines, are a part of the maxillary anatomy known as the

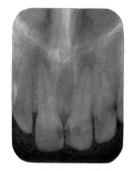

    a. nasal septum
    b. maxillary sinus
    c. nasopalatine foramen
    d. nasal fossae

96. The heavy roentgenopaque shadow overlying the apices of the maxillary molars represents normal anatomy and is called the

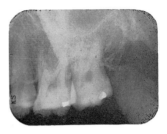

   a. coronoid process of the mandible
   b. zygoma
   c. tuberosity
   d. pterygoid plate

97. The appearance of many small white spots in a scattered pattern on a fully processed film usually is the result of

   a. an unsafe safelight
   b. light leaking into the darkroom
   c. using old film
   d. dirt or dust adhering to the film emulsion

98. The roentgenogram is the result of the roentgen-ray passing through tissues of various densities and registering on the emulsion. Which of the following substances would appear roentgenopaque?

   A. enamel
   B. foramina
   C. nutrient canals
   D. cortical bone
   E. an amalgam restoration

   a. A and B
   b. B and C
   c. A, C, and E
   d. B, C, and D
   e. A, D, and E

99. The operator of dental x-ray equipment must constantly keep in mind the dangers of x-ray to himself and to personnel about him, and maintain between himself and the source of radiation a recommended distance of

   a. a minimum of 6 feet
   b. not less than 2 feet
   c. 4 feet and 45 degrees to the side of the patient
   d. a minimum of four feet

100. Dental roentgenograms may be mounted to view from the buccal or lingual aspects of the teeth. Which of the following factors facilitates mounting?

    A. the embossed dot on the film
    B. normal anatomic landmarks
    C. bone pattern
    D. position of the teeth on the film

    a. A
    b. B and C
    c. A, C, and D
    d. B, C, and D
    e. all of the above

ANSWERS

1. c	26. c	51. e	76. a
2. c	27. a	52. d	77. c
3. e	28. e	53. c	78. e
4. b	29. a	54. b	79. d
5. c	30. b	55. d	80. d
6. e	31. c	56. c	81. d
7. b	32. b	57. c	82. c
8. c	33. a	58. d	83. b
9. a	34. a	59. a	84. c
10. c	35. c	60. b	85. d
11. d	36. c	61. c	86. d
12. c	37. d	62. b	87. b
13. a	38. c	63. c	88. a
14. c	39. c	64. c	89. b
15. c	40. d	65. c	90. b
16. b	41. a	66. b	91. b
17. c	42. c	67. b	92. a
18. a	43. d	68. c	93. c
19. d	44. c	69. b	94. c
20. c	45. b	70. d	95. d
21. d	46. a	71. c	96. b
22. e	47. c	72. a	97. d
23. a	48. d	73. b	98. e
24. b	49. e	74. c	99. a
25. b	50. a	75. c	100. e

REFERENCES

1. Ennis, L. M., Berry, H. M., Jr., and Phillips, J. E.: *Dental Roentgenology*. 6th Ed. Philadelphia, Lea & Febiger, 1967.
2. Wainwright, W. W.: *Dental Radiology*. New York, McGraw-Hill, 1965.
3. Wuehrmann, A. H., and Manson-Hing, L. R.: *Dental Radiology*. St. Louis, C. V. Mosby Co., 1965.

CHAPTER 13

DENTAL PUBLIC HEALTH AND DENTAL HEALTH EDUCATION

Edith R. Sanders

1. The Federal government assumes responsibility for dental care of

    A. indigent persons
    B. physically handicapped persons
    C. persons in Federal institutions
    D. personnel of the Armed Forces

    a. A
    b. A and B
    c. B, C, and D
    d. all of the above

2. Which of the following are characteristics of a group dental practice?

    A. The dentists are equal.
    B. There is a diversity of skills.
    C. All dentists are located in the same building.
    D. The income is pooled.

    a. A and B
    b. A, B, and D
    c. B and D
    d. all of the above

3. Which of the following is characteristic of dental insurance?

    a. It is less expensive than direct payment.
    b. It spreads the cost among all subscribers.
    c. It covers all dental expenses.
    d. all of the above

4. School dental health programs should include provisions for

    a. dental health education
    b. dental care
    c. a healthful environment
    d. all of the above

5. School dental health programs should begin with what age level?

    a. preschool
    b. first grade
    c. third grade
    d. fifth grade

6. In order to provide dental care for the chronically ill, the aged, and the handicapped, a dentist or dental hygienist needs

    a. special equipment
    b. special techniques
    c. special education
    d. all of the above

7. In the event of disaster, dental personnel can aid in

    a. emergency first aid of the injured
    b. training of untrained persons
    c. identification of the dead
    d. all of the above

8. Which of the following are considered acceptable means of financing dental care?

    A. fee-for-service
    B. taxation
    C. prepayment and insurance plans
    D. charity

    a. A
    b. A and C
    c. A, C, and D
    d. all of the above

9. The Department of Welfare in each state provides dental care for

    a. needy persons
    b. unemployed persons
    c. indigent persons
    d. medically indigent persons

10. Which law provides for dental care for the handicapped?

    a. Kerr-Mills
    b. Social Security
    c. Welfare
    d. Economic Opportunity

11. What percentage of the United States population visits the dentist each year?

    a. 30%
    b. 40%
    c. 50%
    d. 60%

12. The dentist-population ratio in the United States is about

    a. 1:500
    b. 1:1000
    c. 1:1500
    d. 1:2000

13. Which areas of the United States have the greatest concentration of dentists?

    a. New England, middle east, and far west
    b. New England, middle west, and far west
    c. New England, middle west, and south
    d. middle west, south west, and far west

14. The optimum dentist population ratio is considered to be about

    a. 1:500
    b. 1:1000
    c. 1:1500
    d. 1:2000

15. In comparison to dentists, the number of auxiliary dental personnel in the United States is

    a. less
    b. the same
    c. slightly more
    d. much greater

16. Comprehensive dental care includes

    a. initial care
    b. maintenance care
    c. neither of the above
    d. both of the above

17. The use of auxiliary personnel by a dentist can increase

    a. his efficiency
    b. his income
    c. the number of patients in his practice
    d. all of the above

18. Dental treatment needs of a group usually are determined on the basis of

    a. dental examinations of the group
    b. the number of persons in the group who visit a dentist each year
    c. the group's demand for dental care
    d. all of the above

19. Demand for dental care is most closely related to a person's

    a. social class
    b. income
    c. education
    d. personality

20. Which one of the following is the most practical solution to the problem of shortage of dentists?

    a. dental health education
    b. free dental clinics
    c. use of preventive dental measures
    d. increased provision of dental benefits by labor unions

21. Dental treatment needs in the United States are equal to approximately how many unfilled cavities?

    a. 1 million
    b. 500 million
    c. 700 million
    d. 1 billion

22. Treatment needs of an individual are determined by the

    A. attack of dental diseases
    B. amount of dental care
    C. demand for dental care
    D. prevalence of dental diseases

    a. A
    b. A and B
    c. A, B, and C
    d. all of the above

23. The most important factor in determining the amount of dental treatment needed by a group is

    a. age
    b. amount of dental diseases
    c. past utilization of dental services
    d. sex

24. Prevalence data for dental diseases are associated with

    a. initial treatment needs for a group
    b. maintenance treatment needs
    c. emergency treatment needs
    d. new treatment needs

25. Treating dental defects as they occur and not waiting until needs build up is called

    a. initial care
    b. groups care
    c. incremental care
    d. essential care

26. Which of the following is related to the utilization of dental services?

    a. needs
    b. desires
    c. demands
    d. all of the above

27. What percentage of the population of the United States utilizes dental services on a routine periodic basis?

    a. 5 to 10%
    b. 15 to 20%
    c. 25 to 30%
    d. 35 to 40%

28. Utilization of dental services varies directly with

    A. age
    B. income
    C. education
    D. amount of dental care

    a. A and B
    b. B and C
    c. C and D
    d. A, B, and C

29. Demand for dental care is related to an individual's

    A. knowledge
    B. attitudes
    C. past dental experience
    D. availability of service

    a. A and B
    b. B
    c. C
    d. all of the above

30. It has been predicted that future demand for dental care will be

    a. greater than at present
    b. less than at present
    c. about the same as at present
    d. considerably less than at present

31. The public health dentist is concerned with the dental health of all

    a. people in the community
    b. people in the neighborhood
    c. school children
    d. indigent people in the community

32. The examination in a dental office can be compared to which aspect of public health dentistry?

    a. analysis
    b. survey
    c. diagnosis
    d. appraisal

33. In public health dentistry, program planning can be compared to which aspect of private dental practice?

    a. treatment
    b. diagnosis
    c. treatment planning
    d. program appraisal

34. Which of the following identifies public health as a specialty within dentistry?

    a. concern for promotion of dental health
    b. concern for dental health of all people
    c. concern for prevention of dental diseases
    d. concern for provision of quality dental care

35. Health practices can be considered to be therapeutic, preventive, and promotive. With which is public health primarily concerned?

    a. preventive
    b. promotive
    c. preventive and therapeutic
    d. preventive and promotive

36. Public health is chiefly concerned with improving the health of

    a. children
    b. everyone
    c. special groups
    d. needy people

37. Prevalence refers to the

    a. cumulative effect of a disease
    b. number of new cases of a disease
    c. rate of disease
    d. proportion of the population affected by a disease

38. The DMF index is a measure of

    a. decayed, missing, and filled teeth
    b. decayed, missing, and filled permanent teeth
    c. decayed, missing, and filled teeth in adults
    d. decayed, missing (or indicated for extraction), and filled permanent teeth

39. The def index is used most accurately with persons aged

    a. 6 and 7 or younger
    b. 8 and 9
    c. 10 and 11
    d. 12 and 13 or older

40. The def index is a measure of

    a. decayed, missing, and filled primary teeth
    b. decayed, extracted, and filled primary teeth
    c. decayed, extracted, and filled teeth
    d. decayed, indicated for extraction because of caries, and filled primary teeth

41. The PMA index is used to measure

    a. dental caries
    b. periodontal disease
    c. gingivitis
    d. oral debris and calculus

42. The PI and PDI indices measure

    a. dental caries
    b. periodontal disease
    c. gingivitis
    d. oral debris and calculus

43. The OHI index is used to measure

    a. dental caries
    b. periodontal disease
    c. gingivitis
    d. oral debris and calculus

44. The arithmetic average used to describe a population is called the

    a. mean
    b. median
    c. mode
    d. module

45. Which of the following denotes the highest correlation between two variables?

    a. $r = .3$
    b. $r = .7$
    c. $r = 7.0$
    d. $r = 30.0$

46. What percentage of people in the United States experience tooth decay?

    a. less than 50%
    b. 50 to 70%
    c. 70 to 90%
    d. 90% or more

47. Studies have shown that there is a definite relation between dental caries and

    A. use of sugar
    B. intake of fluoride
    C. frequency of toothbrushing
    D. adequacy of vitamin C

    a. A and B
    b. A, B, and C
    c. B and C
    d. all of the above

48. Periodontal diseases cause the majority of tooth loss in persons over age

    a. 18
    b. 25
    c. 35
    d. 40

49. Periodontal disease seems to be related most closely to

    a. age
    b. oral hygiene
    c. diet
    d. fluoride

50. Which of the following means of doing a survey is most liable to error?

    a. questionnaire
    b. interview
    c. clinical study
    d. controlled experiment

51. The standard deviation is a measure of

    a. central tendency
    b. variability
    c. significance
    d. correlation

52. Epidemiology is concerned with the

    a. identification of the agent of disease in the host
    b. occurrence and distribution of disease in a population
    c. mutual relation between organisms and their environment
    d. predisposing factors to disease

53. In which of the following ways is the epidemiologic approach useful in controlling disease?

    a. Data can be collected to determine the frequency and distribution of disease.
    b. Hypotheses can be formulated and tested regarding methods for control of disease.
    c. Control measures can be evaluated.
    d. all of the above

54. Dental caries is considered to be what kind of a disease?

    a. acute
    b. infectious
    c. chronic
    d. nutritional — deficiency

55. Which of the following factors seems to have the most effect on whether a person seeks dental care?

    a. socioeconomic status
    b. race
    c. sex
    d. age

56. A survey is useful in

    a. interpreting facts
    b. measuring facts.
    c. collecting facts.
    d. summarizing facts.

57. Current data indicates that persons over age 55 have an average of how many missing teeth?

    a. 10
    b. 15
    c. 20
    d. 25

58. Which of the following is the primary cause of tooth loss among school children?

    a. periodontal diseases
    b. malocclusion
    c. accidents
    d. dental caries

59. Which of the following is the ultimate goal of dental epidemiology?

    a. control of dental diseases
    b. description of dental diseases
    c. identification of dental diseases
    d. development of indices for measuring dental diseases

60. Final proof for the efficacy of fluoridation as a public health measure came at which stage of the epidemiologic investigation?

    a. Dental caries were shown to be related to fluoride consumption.
    b. Fluorosis was shown to be related to drinking water.
    c. Fluoride was identified in water.
    d. Fluoride was successfully added to drinking water in several controlled experiments.

61. Measures for the quantification of dental epidemiologic data are known as
    a. data
    b. numbers
    c. indices
    d. experiences

62. Which of the following is a desirable characteristic for a useful index of dental disease?
    a. reliable
    b. reproducible
    c. practical
    d. all of the above

63. In analyzing scientific data, it is important to determine whether
    a. the sample size is adequate
    b. the sample is representative of the population
    c. any difference shown is a true difference
    d. all of the above

64. Which of the following should be critically considered in evaluating dental literature?
    a. the publication source
    b. the record of the author
    c. the amount of detail used in describing the study
    d. all of the above

65. Which of the following is *not* a function of a state health department's dental division?
    a. research
    b. consultation
    c. education
    d. licensure

66. Federal responsibility for dental health rests with the
    a. Department of Health, Education, and Welfare
    b. National Institutes of Health
    c. Office of Economic Opportunity
    d. National Institute of Dental Health

67. In international dental health, who has primary responsibility?
    a. Pan-American Sanitary Bureau
    b. World Health Organization
    c. International Office of Public Health
    d. United Nations

68. Dental public health programs are administered at which level of government?

    a. federal
    b. state
    c. local
    d. all of the above

69. Which of the following is *not* a function of the federal government in relation to dental health?

    a. consultation
    b. research
    c. administration of local programs
    d. education

70. Which of the following activities of dental public health at the community level has a part in almost all other activities?

    a. professional development
    b. research
    c. education
    d. remedial treatment

71. Dental programs for the prevention of dental diseases usually are administered at which level of dental public health?

    a. local
    b. state
    c. federal
    d. all of the above

72. Which of the following is primarily a function of the state level of dental public health?

    a. periodic examination of children's teeth in a school system
    b. research in methods for detecting oral cancer
    c. consultation to teachers concerning dental health
    d. conducting a school's dental health day

73. A disease is considered a public health problem if

    a. the disease is widespread
    b. knowledge exists about how to prevent, cure, or alleviate the disease
    c. knowledge about how to prevent, cure, or alleviate the disease is not being applied effectively and efficiently
    d. all of the above

74. The most important responsibility of the dental division of a state health department is to
    a. distribute dental health educational materials
    b. provide free dental treatment to indigent children
    c. provide consultation in dental health matters
    d. provide funds to establish community dental health programs

75. Many people would consider the primary role of the dental hygienist in the dental office to be
    a. prophylaxis
    b. education
    c. examination
    d. diagnosis

76. A dental hygienist can provide leadership in a community by
    A. promoting fluoridation
    B. teaching correct dental health habits
    C. continuing her education
    D. belonging to her professional organization

    a. A
    b. A and B
    c. A, B, and D
    d. all of the above

77. A dental hygienist should take an active part in dental health education in which of the following areas?
    a. the home
    b. the schools
    c. the community in general
    d. all of the above

78. A dental hygienist should participate in community programs for prevention of dental diseases because
    a. the efforts of the dentist and the dental hygienist in the private dental office cannot benefit everyone
    b. dental diseases are a major health problem
    c. effective preventive measures exist for the control of dental diseases
    d. all of the above

79. For which of the following reasons should a dentist or dental hygienist participate in community dental health programs?
    a. to save effort
    b. to save time
    c. to meet dental needs of the community
    d. all of the above

80. To promote fluoridation in a community, a dentist or dental hygienist may have to assume the role of

     a. leader
     b. politician
     c. expert
     d. all of the above

81. To ensure success in gaining fluoridation for a community, a dentist or dental hygienist should

     a. work with known leaders in the community
     b. identify themselves as leaders in a campaign for fluoridation
     c. compete publicly with politicians
     d. call attention to themselves as active supporters of fluoridation

82. Which is the ideal method of gaining fluoridation for a community?

     a. referendum
     b. public vote
     c. decision of elected representatives of the public
     d. decision of leaders of the community

83. School dental inspections are considered by some people to be a waste of time for dental personnel. Why?

     a. It is a known fact that 90% or more school children need dental care.
     b. Dental inspections are only cursory and may give parents a false sense of security if no obvious defects are present.
     c. Time doing dental inspections could be spent more profitably doing dental treatment.
     d. all of the above

84. When might a dental hygienist sensibly participate in mass dental inspections of school children?

     a. for research purposes
     b. for purposes of evaluation
     c. for estimating treatment needs
     d. all of the above

85. It is the responsibility of the dentist and dental hygienist to recommend to schools that

     a. athletes should wear mouthguards
     b. sale of candy and sweetened beverages should be abolished
     c. dental health should be taught as a regular part of the total health curriculum
     d. all of the above

86. A dental hygienist when employed in a school system will function best by
    a. instructing all classes in dental health
    b. doing oral inspections
    c. constructing visual aids
    d. acting as a resource person for teachers

87. Strong community programs for dental health are primarily the result of
    a. coordinated interest and effort of citizens and professional persons
    b. quantity and quality of professional personnel
    c. strength of the health department
    d. strength of the school health program

88. Which of the following activities would be suitable for a dental hygienist in a school dental health program?
    A. helping teachers with dental health teaching
    B. serving as a member of the school health council
    C. conducting dental inspections of school children
    D. performing prophylaxes and topical applications of fluoride

    a. A, B, and C
    b. A, B, and D
    c. A, C, and D
    d. all of the above

89. Which of the following is related to the ability of a dentist and dental hygienist to provide the best service to the public?
    A. location of the office
    B. use of auxiliary personnel
    C. continuation of their education
    D. utilization of preventive services

    a. A
    b. B and D
    c. B, C, and D
    d. all of the above

90. In assuming some responsibility for the oral health of the handicapped, chronically ill, and aged, the dentist and dental hygienist should be prepared to
    a. perform needed services for such people who come to the office
    b. work with people in the community to see that such persons receive needed dental care
    c. function in both capacities as indicated above
    d. function in neither capacity as indicated above

91. If a dental hygienist is invited to speak on dental health to a group of nurses, she should

    a. decline the invitation saying that a dentist could do it better
    b. go ahead and make the speech
    c. make the speech after preparing herself adequately
    d. consult with the local dental society and then make the speech with adequate preparation

92. Health promotion and specific protection are considered to occur at which level of prevention?

    a. primary
    b. secondary
    c. tertiary
    d. all three levels

93. Fluoridation is an example of which level of prevention?

    a. primary
    b. secondary
    c. tertiary
    d. all three levels

94. Examinations of the teeth of school children exemplify which level of prevention?

    a. primary
    b. secondary
    c. tertiary
    d. all three levels

95. Toothbrushing appears to be most effective in the prevention of

    a. dental caries
    b. malocclusion
    c. periodontal diseases
    d. bad breath

96. A prophylaxis is most helpful in the prevention of

    a. dental caries
    b. malocclusion
    c. periodontal diseases
    d. all of the above

97. The occurrence of dental caries is closely related to

    A. frequency of toothbrushing
    B. amount of sugar consumed
    C. frequency of eating sweets
    D. frequency of dental prophylaxis

    a. A and B
    b. D
    c. B and C
    d. all of the above

98. Which of the following would be the best substitutions for sweets between meals?

    a. sugarless gum, apples, popcorn
    b. fresh fruits, graham crackers, nuts
    c. sugarless gum, nuts, popcorn
    d. fresh fruits, raisins, nuts

99. Tooth decay can be reduced through the dietary control of

    a. fermentable carbohydrates
    b. fats
    c. protein
    d. vitamins

100. Which of the following is the best method for the prevention of tooth decay?

    a. toothbrushing
    b. restriction of sweets
    c. fluoridation
    d. topical application of fluoride

101. Which of the following ways of using fluoride is most effective in reducing tooth decay?

    a. fluoridation
    b. topical application
    c. fluoride toothpaste
    d. fluoride in vitamin pills

102. Which of the following is indicative of the amount of dental caries activity?

    a. lactobacillus count
    b. Snyder test
    c. both of the above
    d. neither of the above

103. Malocclusion often can be prevented by

    a. use of space maintainers
    b. replacement of missing teeth
    c. control of thumbsucking
    d. all of the above

104. Oral cancer can be prevented most effectively by

    a. early recognition
    b. biopsy
    c. treatment
    d. referral

105. Mouthguards to prevent accidents to teeth are most practical for

    a. all children
    b. all persons engaged in contact sports
    c. automobile passengers
    d. persons on organized athletic teams

106. In groups of children who drink fluoridated water from birth, tooth decay can be reduced by as much as

    a. 40%
    b. 50%
    c. 60%
    d. 80%

107. Which of the following nutrients is helpful in the prevention of tooth decay?

    a. calcium
    b. vitamin C
    c. fluoride
    d. all of the above

108. The adjustment of fluoride in a water supply to the optimum amount is related to

    a. climate.
    b. mean annual temperature.
    c. water consumption
    d. humidity

109. The annual cost of fluoridation per person is said to be approximately

    a. 10 cents
    b. $1.00
    c. $10.00
    d. $100.00

110. Parents should be urged to begin taking children to a dentist at age

    a. three
    b. five
    c. six
    d. eight

111. Dental hygienists can be utilized most effectively at which levels of prevention?

    a. primary and secondary
    b. primary and tertiary
    c. secondary and tertiary
    d. all three levels

112. Fluoridation is an ideal public health measure because it is

    a. devoid of hazard to life or function
    b. effective immediately and over a long period of time in reaching all people in a community
    c. available at a cost in money and facilities within the economic capabilities of a community
    d. all of the above

113. If fluoridation is impractical in a community, which of the following would be considered acceptable?

    a. topical applications of fluoride
    b. dietary supplements of fluoride
    c. fluoridation of school water supplies
    d. all of the above

114. Topical application of stannous fluoride has been reported to reduce tooth decay by as much as

    a. 40%
    b. 50%
    c. 60%
    d. 80%

115. Topical application of sodium fluoride will reduce tooth decay by about

    a. 40%
    b. 50%
    c. 60%
    d. 80%

116. Which of the following is *not* considered particularly important in the prevention of tooth decay?

    a. fluoridation
    b. toothbrushing
    c. diet
    d. regular dental care

117. Which of the following is *not* considered very important in prevention of periodontal diseases?

    a. fluoridation
    b. toothbrushing
    c. diet
    d. regular dental care

118. Which of the following would be considered a preventive measure in the dental office?

    A. education
    B. prophylaxis
    C. restoration
    D. recall

    a. A and B
    b. A and C
    c. A, B, and D
    d. all of the above

119. Which of the following are considered valuable as preventive dental measures for a community?

    A. adjustment of fluoride content of drinking water
    B. screening for dental defects
    C. topical applications of fluoride
    D. provision of mouthguards for athletes

    a. A
    b. B
    c. B and C
    d. all of the above

120. In what way does a dental survey aid in a preventive program?

    a. identifies problems of a community
    b. suggests ways to attack problems of a community
    c. aids in evaluation of program
    d. all of the above

121. The ultimate responsibility for the prevention and control of dental diseases rests with

     a. public health agencies
     b. schools
     c. dentists
     d. parents

122. At the present time, which method of toothbrushing seems to show the most promise in effective removal of oral debris?

     a. Bass method
     b. brushing the teeth the way they grow
     c. using a disclosing wafer and brushing until the teeth are clean
     d. modified Charter's method

123. If the existing fluoride content of a water supply were 0.3 ppm, usually what amount would be added to have an optimum amount?

     a. 0.7 ppm
     b. 1.0 ppm
     c. 1.2 ppm
     d. 1.7 ppm

124. Which of the following programs should receive priority as a dental public health measure?

     a. topical fluoride clinics
     b. dental care programs for children
     c. promotion of fluoridation
     d. dental health education in schools

125. When in the educational process should evaluation be used?

     a. at the beginning
     b. at the end
     c. about half way through
     d. continually

126. In modern educational theory, learning is best compared to which of the following?

     a. listening
     b. changing
     c. thinking
     d. recalling

127. Education is useful at which level of prevention?

    a. primary
    b. secondary
    c. tertiary
    d. all three levels

128. Which of the following usually is the most effective means of education?

    a. mass media
    b. distribution of pamphlets
    c. individual instruction
    d. lecture

129. In order to accomplish their purpose, dental health educational materials ideally should be

    a. based on accurate scientific information
    b. easy to read by the age group for which they are designed
    c. attractive and eye-catching in relation to color and layout used
    d. all of the above

130. Which of the following is the superior method for dental health education?

    a. a dentist lecturing about teeth in a classroom
    b. a dental hygienist lecturing about teeth in a classroom
    c. a teacher incorporating dental health teaching into the regular classroom instruction
    d. a health educator lecturing on dental health in a classroom

131. Dental health education is considered an important part of health education because

    A. dental diseases are almost universally prevalent
    B. dental diseases can be partially prevented
    C. teeth are important physiologically
    D. teeth are important esthetically

    a. A and B
    b. A and C
    c. A, B, and C
    d. all of the above

132. A comprehensive school dental health program should consist of

    a. provisions for dental care
    b. dental health instruction
    c. an optimum environment for the prevention of accidents to teeth
    d. all of the above

133. The responsibility for dental health rests *primarily* with the

    a. individual
    b. family
    c. community
    d. state.

134. Dental health educational programs, in order to be successful, require the cooperation of people in

    a. the home and the school
    b. the school and the community
    c. the home and the community
    d. the home, the school, and the community

135. In order to be effective, dental health teaching must enable the learner to

    a. learn all the facts about teeth
    b. memorize the parts of a tooth.
    c. cultivate desirable dental attitudes and habits
    d. know all of the above

136. Dental health education should be related to the individual's

    A. needs
    B. past experiences
    C. interests
    D. economic status

    a. A and B
    b. A and C
    c. A, B, and C
    d. all of the above

137. Present concepts in health education emphasize

    a. treatment
    b. instruction
    c. knowledge
    d. activity

138. Visual aids are useful

    a. to supplement one's teaching
    b. to use instead of a lecture.
    c. to educate patients while they are waiting
    d. for all the above reasons.

139. Which of the following is most likely to lead to learning?

      a. participating in an experience
      b. watching a film
      c. dramatizing a situation
      d. reading a textbook

140. Which of the following are desirable traits for a group discussion leader?

      A. controls the members of the group
      B. releases the flow of conversation after starting it
      C. dominates the discussion
      D. suppresses overly talkative members of the group

      a. B
      b. B and C
      c. A, B, and D
      d. all of the above

141. To be a successful member of a group discussion one should be

      A. informed.
      B. talkative
      C. cooperative
      D. neutral

      a. A and B
      b. B and C
      c. A and D
      d. A and C

142. Which of the following is likely to be a basis for motivating adults to be interested in dental health?

      a. their future dental health
      b. their immediate dental needs
      c. the cost of dental care
      d. all of the above

143. The most effective means of coordinating a dental health program with the total health program in a community is through a

      a. parent teacher association
      b. dental health committee
      c. community health council
      d. health department

144. Visual aids in the dental office will be most effective if they are

    a. displayed prominently in the office
    b. used for "shock" value.
    c. used to illustrate specific points when talking with a patient
    d. all of the above

145. Dental health pamphlets are most useful if they are

    a. sent through the mail to the dentist's patients
    b. left in the reception room of the dental office
    c. distributed to large audiences when making a talk on dental health.
    d. given to individuals in response to a specific question

146. The evaluation of a dental health program in schools should be concerned primarily with the

    a. number of teeth filled
    b. number of teeth extracted
    c. reaction of professional persons to the program
    d. ability of the program to reduce dental diseases

147. Routine dental inspections of school children are of little value unless

    a. a parent is present
    b. a diagnosis is made
    c. they are done at least once a year
    d. they result in children obtaining needed dental care

148. Which of the following are aims and objectives for a school dental health program according to the American Dental Association?

    A. to help every child appreciate the importance of a complete set of teeth and a healthy mouth
    B. to show the relationship of dental health to general health
    C. to provide needed dental care for all children of school age
    D. to enlist the cooperation of parents in these efforts to obtain adequate dental care

    a. A and B
    b. A, B, and C
    c. A, B, and D
    d. all of the above

149. A dental health service program in a school might include

    a. periodic dental inspections
    b. records of dental health status
    c. informing parents of dental defects
    d. all of the above

150. Children are most likely to show interest in dental health because of concern for

    a. their future dental health
    b. the cost of dental treatment
    c. their immediate problems
    d. the efficiency of their chewing

151. Which of the following criteria is most essential in the selection of dental health educational materials?

    a. attractive illustrations
    b. authentic content
    c. attractive color combinations
    d. suitable literary style

152. Which of the following is the best measure of effective dental health education?

    a. application of knowledge to daily living
    b. high score on a dental health quiz
    c. an extensive community program during National Children's Dental Health Week
    d. the number of dental health films shown annually in a school

153. The use of mass media in dental health education is

    a. equally effective for all groups
    b. effective in gaining a specific response
    c. limited in its effectiveness to influence behavior
    d. effective in reaching the group one desires to reach

154. Which of the following have a bearing on dental health education in the dental office?

    A. the way the telephone is answered
    B. what the reception room looks like
    C. how well the patient and dentist understand each other
    D. the concern of the dentist and dental hygienist for the patient

    a. C and D
    b. B, C, and D
    c. D only
    d. all of the above

155. Why does a dental hygienist have a greater opportunity than the dentist to provide dental health education in the dental office?

    a. She rarely performs a painful procedure.
    b. She is trained in educational methods.
    c. She often has the first contact with a patient in the dental office
    d. all of the above

156. In preparing a dental health educational program for a school, what is the first thing that should be done?

    a. Find out what is being taught already.
    b. Conduct an in-service dental health educational program for the teachers.
    c. Distribute to all teachers the ADA booklet, "Dental Health Facts for Teachers."
    d. Ask commercial organizations for help in conducting the program.

157. When should a dental hygienist participate in direct classroom instruction concerning dental health?

    a. when the class has been working on a project on dental health
    b. when students have questions the teacher cannot answer
    c. when the teacher feels that they would benefit from having a guest expert come into the classroom
    d. in all of the above situations

158. Instead of providing direct classroom instruction, dentists and dental hygienists can spend their time in schools more wisely in

    a. providing consultation for teachers
    b. helping to prepare educational materials
    c. reviewing textbooks
    d. all of the above

159. In addition to schools, other community outlets for dental health information include

    a. other professional groups
    b. well child conferences
    c. career days
    d. all of the above

160. Which of the following resources might be available at the local level for help in dental health programs?

    A. community health council
    B. voluntary agencies
    C. health department
    D. civic organizations

    a. C only
    b. B and C
    c. A, C, and D
    d. all of the above

161. At the state level, where would help be available for planning a community dental health program?

    a. dental association
    b. health department
    c. department of public education
    d. all of the above

162. The dental service corporation can be compared to

    a. Medicare
    b. group practice
    c. Blue Cross–Blue Shield plans
    d. commercial insurance companies

163. The source of funds in a dental care plan may be from

    A. the patients
    B. an employer
    C. a governmental agency
    D. a dental society

    a. A and B
    b. A and C
    c. A, B, and C
    d. all of the above

164. Payment of dentists in a dental care program may be

    a. a salary
    b. on a per capita basis
    c. payment for service
    d. any of the above methods

165. Which of the following would be considered a desirable characteristic of dental service corporations?

    a. Negotiations take place between organizations
    b. The individual dentist does not have to bargain for himself concerning fees
    c. The patients do not have to determine for themselves the quality and value of services.
    d. all of the above

166. Which of the following is the test of the value of a dental care plan?

    a. its ability to extend dental service of high quality to more people
    b. the number of patients that can be seen yearly
    c. its ability to keep fees low
    d. the number of patients who keep their teeth for a lifetime

167. The supply of dentists in a specific area is related to

    a. average per capita income
    b. educational level
    c. the percentage of rural population
    d. all of the above

168. Which of the following holds the most promise in meeting future demands for dental care?

    a. reducing dental needs through such measures as fluoridation
    b. increasing the supply of dentists
    c. increasing productivity through use of auxiliary personnel
    d. developing an extensive dental health educational program

169. According to behavioral scientists, which of the following conditions must exist before a person will take action to regain or preserve his health?

    a. a feeling of susceptibility to a certain disease or condition
    b. a feeling that the disease or condition would be severe if it occurred
    c. a feeling that there is an action that can be taken to reduce the susceptibility or severity of the condition
    d. all of the above

170. The development of dental health programs must take into account

    a. motivation of individuals
    b. sufficiency of funds
    c. careful selection of objectives
    d. all of the above

171. The percentage of dental practices that are considered moderately or highly preventive is about

    a. 50%
    b. 60%
    c. 70%
    d. 80% or more

172. The majority of dental hygienists spend how much of their time in patient education?

    a. less than 30%
    b. 50%
    c. 75%
    d. 80% or more

173. What is the major role of the teacher in dental health education?

    a. to lecture to students about dental health
    b. to provide sufficient dental health educational materials
    c. to guide students' behavior in the desirable direction
    d. to direct them to the dentist for needed dental care

174. At what time in the process of satisfying a need does a person learn?

    a. before acting to satisfy the need
    b. between the time the need is realized and it is acted upon
    c. while acting to satisfy the need
    d. after the need is satisfied

175. Dental diseases are considered public health problems because

    A. they are widespread
    B. civic leaders recognize them
    C. knowledge exists to prevent them
    D. methods for prevention are not being fully applied

    a. A and C
    b. B and D
    c. A, C and D
    d. D only

ANSWERS

1. d	21. c	41. c	61. c
2. d	22. c	42. b	62. d
3. b	23. c	43. d	63. d
4. d	24. a	44. a	64. d
5. a	25. c	45. b	65. d
6. d	26. d	46. d	66. a
7. d	27. b	47. a	67. b
8. d	28. b	48. c	68. d
9. c	29. d	49. b	69. c
10. b	30. a	50. a	70. c
11. b	31. a	51. b	71. a
12. d	32. b	52. b	72. c
13. a	33. c	53. d	73. d
14. b	34. b	54. c	74. c
15. d	35. d	55. a	75. b
16. d	36. b	56. c	76. d
17. d	37. d	57. c	77. d
18. a	38. d	58. d	78. d
19. c	39. a	59. a	79. d
20. c	40. d	60. d	80. d

81. a	105. d	129. d	153. c
82. c	106. c	130. c	154. d
83. d	107. c	131. d	155. d
84. d	108. b	132. d	156. a
85. d	109. a	133. a	157. d
86. d	110. a	134. d	158. d
87. a	111. a	135. c	159. d
88. d	112. d	136. d	160. d
89. d	113. d	137. d	161. d
90. c	114. d	138. a	162. c
91. d	115. a	139. a	163. c
92. a	116. b	140. c	164. d
93. a	117. a	141. d	165. d
94. b	118. d	142. d	166. a
95. c	119. d	143. c	167. d
96. c	120. d	144. c	168. c
97. c	121. d	145. d	169. d
98. c	122. c	146. d	170. d
99. a	123. a	147. d	171. a
100. c	124. c	148. c	172. a
101. a	125. d	149. d	173. c
102. c	126. b	150. c	174. c
103. d	127. d	151. b	175. c
104. a	128. c	152. a	

REFERENCES

1. Dunning, J. M.: *Principles of Dental Public Health*. Cambridge, Harvard University Press, 1962.
2. Hollinshead, B. S.: *The Survey of Dentistry,* The Final Report, Washington, D.C., The American Council on Education, 1961.
3. Podshadley, D. W., and Weiss, R. L.: *Introduction to Dental Public Health,* A Self-Instruction Course. Washington, D.C., Government Printing Office, 1964.
4. Steele, P. F.: *Dimensions of Dental Hygiene*. Philadelphia, Lea & Febiger, 1966.
5. Stoll, F. A., and Catherman, J.: *Dental Health Education,* 3rd Ed. Philadelphia, Lea & Febiger, 1967.
6. Young, W. O., and Striffler, D. F.: *The Dentist, His Practice, and His Community*. Philadelphia, W. B. Saunders Co., 1964.

CHAPTER 14

DENTAL HYGIENE HISTORY, ORGANIZATION, JURISPRU-DENCE, AND OFFICE ADMINISTRATION

Pauline F. Steele

1. The dental hygienist utilizes dental x-rays for

    a. diagnostic purposes
    b. therapeutic purposes
    c. evaluative purposes
    d. none of the above

2. Dr. W. D. Miller's theory of dental caries was premised upon the theory of

    a. chemo-biologic agents
    b. chemo-bacteriologic agents
    c. chemo-parasitic agents
    d. chemo-therapeutic agents

3. X-rays were discovered in the

    a. twenty-first century
    b. twentieth century
    c. nineteenth century
    d. eighteenth century

4. The precise cause of dental decay has been under investigation for many years, but it is now

    a. firmly established
    b. seldom under research
    c. still being investigated
    d. both a and b

5. The specialty of exodontia involves

    a. all oral surgery procedures
    b. only extractions
    c. just surgical procedures
    d. all of the above

6. Periodontal disease affects

    a. only adults
    b. few children
    c. usually youth
    d. all segments of the population

7. The dental hygienist in some instances is allowed to administer anesthetics that are

    a. local
    b. topical
    c. general
    d. parenteral

8. The individual who organized the idea of placing anesthetic solutions in a cartridge was

    a. Harvey S. Cook
    b. Horace Wells
    c. J. F. Simpson
    d. W. G. Morten

9. Operative dental techniques were perfected by

    a. John M. Riggs
    b. Thomas Fillebrown
    c. C. Edmund Kells
    d. G. V. Black

10. The practice of orthodontics was systematized through the efforts of

    a. Norman W. Ringsley
    b. Edward H. Angle
    c. William H. Taggart
    d. Crawford W. Long

11. The patron saint of dentistry is

    a. St. Cosmos
    b. St. Damos
    c. St. Appolonia
    d. St. Francis

12. A term that describes trial and error method is

    a. emperical
    b. scientific
    c. experimental
    d. none of the above

13. The first dental college to be established was known as the

    a. Ohio College of Dental Surgery
    b. Philadelphia College of Dental Surgery
    c. Baltimore College of Dental Surgery
    d. Pennsylvania College of Dental Surgery

14. The first dental periodical was entitled

    a. Dental Newsletter
    b. Dental Cosmos
    c. American Journal of Dental Science
    d. Journal of the National Dental Association

15. The first dental hygiene textbook was entitled

    a. Oral Hygiene
    b. Dental Hygiene
    c. Mouth Hygiene
    d. none of the above

16. The first dental hygiene textbook was edited by

    a. A. C. Fones
    b. R. W. Strang
    c. E. C. Kirk
    d. Russell Bunting

17. The specialty of prosthodontics is restricted to the fabrication of

    a. dentures
    b. dentures and speech appliances
    c. dentures, speech appliances, and crowns
    d. dentures and crowns

18. Dental decay has existed since the beginning of

    a. modern civilization
    b. ancient civilization
    c. medieval civilization
    d. Arabian civilization

19. Early dentistry characteristically emphasized

    a. prevention
    b. restoration
    c. cure
    d. all of the above

20. Advertising of services by practicing members of the dental profession is

    a. illegal and forbidden in all forms
    b. a breach of ethical principles
    c. restricted to specialists
    d. a legally and professionally approved procedure if practiced with moderation and discretion

21. Odontalgia is synonymous with the term

    a. extraction
    b. toothache
    c. toothless
    d. dentition

22. The word etiology means

    a. source
    b. cause
    c. origin
    d. all of these

23. The study of gingival conditions is known as

    a. periodontitis
    b. periodontosis
    c. periodontium
    d. periodontics

24. Osseous tissue is more commonly described as

    a. blood
    b. bone
    c. brain
    d. none of these

25. The discoverer of x-rays was

    a. C. Edmund Kells
    b. Horace Wells
    c. E. Rynde
    d. W. K. Roentgen

26. The "father of dental education" was

    a. Chapin Harris
    b. John Harris
    c. Edward Hudson
    d. William Halstead

27. The technical term denoting an abscess of the gingiva is

    a. canker
    b. aphthae
    c. parulis
    d. epulis

28. Much of early dentistry was practiced by

    a. resident dentists
    b. itinerant dentists
    c. specializing dentists
    d. group dentists

29. Dental schools with programs designed for monetary reasons only were called

    a. purveyor
    b. proponent
    c. preceptor
    d. proprietary

30. The dental hygienist must work under the direction of a

    a. graduate dentist
    b. registered dentist
    c. reputable dentist
    d. respectable dentist

31. The services of the dental hygienist are

    a. therapeutic
    b. curative
    c. preventive
    d. restorative

32. Interest in organized dental hygiene programs developed during the

    a. seventeenth century
    b. eighteenth century
    c. nineteenth century
    d. twentieth century

33. The employment trend indicates that the majority of practicing dental hygienists enter

    a. public health
    b. teaching
    c. private practice
    d. research

34. Currently the ratio of dental hygienists to dentists is

    a. 6 to 1
    b. 8 to 1
    c. 10 to 1
    d. 12 to 1

35. In the 1964 Survey of Dentist Opinion, it was disclosed that the major reason presented for not employing a dental hygienist was

    a. too expensive
    b. not available
    c. patient nonacceptance
    d. dentist reluctance

36. The last state to license the dental hygienist was

    a. Illinois
    b. Idaho
    c. Texas
    d. none of the above

37. In the United States, all dental hygiene programs must be a minimum of

    a. one calendar year
    b. one academic year
    c. two calendar years
    d. two academic years

38. The practicing dental hygienist must be licensed in

    a. the state of residence
    b. the state of employment
    c. the state of graduation
    d. all of the above

39. The "father of dental hygiene" was

    a. D. D. Smith
    b. James W. Smith
    c. A. C. Fones
    d. C. M. Wright

40. The appointed officers of the American Dental Hygienists' Association are the

    a. President, Executive Secretary, and Treasurer
    b. President, Journal Editor, and Treasurer
    c. President, Executive Secretary, and Journal Editor
    d. Executive Secretary, Treasurer, and Journal Editor

41. A constituent organization is identical to a

    a. local society
    b. district society
    c. state society
    d. regional society

42. Author of the Dental Hygienists Oath was

    a. J. T. Fulton
    b. Thomas Hunter
    c. Frank Lamons
    d. J. W. Knutson

43. The first dental hygienist with Project Hope was

    a. Christina King
    b. Doris Winter
    c. Jacqueline Huot
    d. Julia Wehrle

44. The first recognized dental hygienist was

    a. Irene Newman
    b. V. M. Createn
    c. M. Freeman Wallis
    d. none of the above

45. Accreditation requirements stipulate that dental hygiene programs be

    a. associated with a dental school
    b. a department of a university
    c. a part of an institute of higher learning
    d. incorporated with a university discipline

46. The National Board of Dental Hygiene Examinations is presently accepted by

    a. all state boards of dental examiners
    b. more than half of all state boards of dental examiners
    c. less than half of all state boards of dental examiners
    d. few state boards of dental examiners

47. The dental hygiene profession is represented on the National Board of Dental Examiners through the Committee on Dental Hygiene by

    a. two dental hygienists
    b. three dental hygienists
    c. four dental hygienists
    d. five dental hygienists

48. Currently there is recognized reciprocity for the dental hygienist in

    a. more than half of all the states
    c. less than half of all the states
    c. all states
    d. most states

49. All states have recognized licensure of the dental hygienist since the year

    a. 1921
    b. 1931
    c. 1941
    d. 1951

50. Dental hygiene laws are characteristically

    a. universal in acceptance by states
    b. non-universal in acceptance by states
    c. generally universal in acceptance by states
    d. commonly universal in acceptance by states

51. The original school for dental hygienists appeared in the year

    a. 1903
    b. 1913
    c. 1923
    d. 1933

52. Recognition of a dental hygienist's license is

    a. a matter of federal regulation
    b. a matter of individual state law
    c. regulated by the National Dental Hygiene Board
    d. discretionary with each state's dental examining board

53. Recognized experimental programs attempting to broaden the scope of services for the dental hygienist have been

    a. met with complete failure
    b. accepted with enthusiasm
    c. accepted with reluctance
    d. met with considerable success

54. Reciprocity for dental hygiene licensure is

    a. actively sought by state licensing boards
    b. seldom advocated by the licensing authority
    c. of little or no concern to the practicing hygienist
    d. basically undesirable

55. Junior membership was incorporated as a segment of the American Dental Hygienists' Association in the year

    a. 1917
    b. 1927
    c. 1937
    d. 1947

56. Statutes governing the licensure and practice of dental hygiene are

    a. usually specific in nature
    b. most frequently general in nature
    c. comprehensive in their coverage
    d. often vague and subject to extensive interpretation

57. State dental hygiene licensure examinations are given by a

    a. special dental hygiene board
    b. special dental board
    c. regular dental board
    d. regular dental hygiene board

58. The duration of a license to practice dental hygiene is usually

    a. for the lifetime of the licensee
    b. for a specified term of years
    c. issued subject to conditions for continuance
    d. subject to annual renewal

59. The American Dental Hygienists' Association is organized into the following units of

    a. constituents, states, and components
    b. components, locals, and districts
    c. constituents, components, and states
    d. components, constituents, and districts

60. A component organization is identical to a

    a. local society
    b. district society
    c. state society
    d. regional society

61. The National Board of Dental Hygiene Examinations Certificate requires

    a. renewal to remain in effect
    b. reporting change of employment
    c. annual reporting of employment
    d. none of the above

62. The American Dental Hygienists' Association House of Delegates is the

    a. appointed body
    b. judicial body
    c. legislative body
    d. executive body

63. The original dental hygiene practice act was proposed by

    a. M. L. Rhein
    b. A. C. Fones
    c. C. M. Wright
    d. E. C. Kirk

64. The National Board of Dental Hygiene Examinations has been in existence since the year

    a. 1932
    b. 1942
    c. 1952.
    d. 1962

65. The first state to license the dental hygienist was

    a. New York.
    b. Massachusetts
    c. Connecticut
    d. none of the above

66. The district trustee of the American Dental Hygienists' Association is

    b. a regional officer
    b. a state officer
    c. a national officer
    d. all of the above

67. The first constituent organization for the dental hygienist appeared in

    a. 1905.
    b. 1915
    c. 1925
    d. 1935

68. The male hygienist is permitted to practice in

   a. many states
   b. few states.
   c. no states
   d. all states

69. Reciprocity licensure is the responsibility of

   a. National Dental Hygiene Board
   b. state dental board to which the application is addressed
   c. Commission on Uniform State Laws
   d. American Dental Health Association

70. The Board of Trustees of the American Dental Hygienists' Association functions in

   a. an executive capacity
   b. a legislative capacity
   c. a judicial capacity
   d. an elective capacity

71. The voting privilege of the American Dental Hygienists' Association Board resides with

   a. all officers
   b. only elected officers
   c. only appointed officers
   d. only special officers

72. The first full time executive secretary of the American Dental Hygienists' Association was

   a. Rebekah Fisk
   b. Mildred Gilsdorf
   c. Ethel Covington
   d. Margaret E. Swanson

73. Central office of the American Dental Hygienists' Association was originally located in

   a. Chicago, Illinois
   b. Cleveland, Ohio
   c. Washington, D. C.
   d. none of the above

74. The male applicant for dental hygiene study is accepted in

   a. all dental hygiene programs
   b. many dental hygiene programs
   c. few dental hygiene programs
   d. several dental hygiene programs

75. The official accrediting agency for any dental hygiene curriculum is the

    a. American Dental Hygienists' Association
    b. American Association of Dental Schools.
    c. American Association of Dental Examiners
    d. American Dental Association

76. The accrediting program for dental hygiene curriculums has been in existence since the year

    a. 1932
    b. 1942
    c. 1952.
    d. 1962

77. The accrediting committee members are comprised of

    a. only dentists
    b. only dental hygienists
    c. several dentists and a dental hygienist representative
    d. several hygienists and a dental representative

78. The laws governing the licensing of dental hygienists and the practice of dental hygiene are characteristically

    a. uniform in the several states
    b. unique to each of the several states
    c. in conformity to federal standards
    d. of a general pattern but not uniform in the several states

79. The dental hygienist is obligated to notify the state board of dental examiners of

    a. change of employment within a state
    b. change of state residence
    c. change of local address
    d. all of the above

80. Auxiliary dental personnel may be guilty of malpractice if

    a. they fail to use the dentist's standard of care
    b. they cause injury to the patient
    c. they fail to use the standard of care current in the community for such services
    d. they fail to adhere to the standards of ethical practice established by the state dental board

81. Certification of a check means that the

    a. bank agrees to honor the check when it is presented for payment
    b. drawer of the check has an account with the bank
    c. amount of the check is verified
    d. check is negotiable

82. In reconciling a monthly bank statement of account, an outstanding check must be considered as the equivalent of a

    a. cancelled check
    b. certified check
    c. verified check
    d. delinquent check

83. Jurisprudence relates to

    a. the science of law
    b. a system of laws
    c. a department of law
    d. all of the above

84. Ethics pertains to

    a. abiding within the law
    b. adhering to a professional code
    c. respecting the rights of others
    d. religious principles

85. The capital value of a dental practice is ascertained as being solvent by determining that the

    a. liabilities exceed the assets
    b. assets exceed the liabilities
    c. charges exceed the liabilities
    d. expenses exceed the assets

86. A check is endorsed when the payee puts his name on the check for the purpose of

    a. depositing the check
    b. identifying himself
    c. negotiating the check
    d. protesting the check

87. An invoice is a statement

    a. demanding payment
    b. describing purchases
    c. approving payment
    d. approving purchases

88. A monthly statement reveals

    a. the balance currently due
    b. the charges made during the previous month
    c. the credits given during the previous month
    d. all of the above

89. The process of bringing about an agreement between the cash balance as shown in the bank statement and the balance as shown in the check book is known as

    a. accreditation
    b. verification
    c. reconciliation
    d. certification

90. An effective recall system utilizes

    a. a double-index system
    b. a cross-index system
    c. an alphabetical index system
    d. a numerical index system

91. Before issuing a license to a dental hygienist, state board examiners require evidence of proficiency in

    a. only clinical or technical information
    b. only academic or theoretical information
    c. both clinical and academic information
    d. either clinical or academic information

92. The dental hygienist is permitted to practice with a temporary license by

    a. all state boards of dental examiners
    b. no state board of dental examiners
    c. more than half of the state boards of dental examiners
    d. less than half of the state boards of dental examiners

93. State board licensure for the dental hygienist must be renewed

    a. annually
    b. periodically
    c. semiannually
    d. biannually

94. It would be against the law for any one dentist to employ more than

    a. one dental hygienist
    b. two dental hygienists
    c. three dental hygienists
    d. four dental hygienists

95. State boards of dental examiners are usually

    a. appointed to office by the state governor
    b. elected to office by the state dental association
    c. appointed to office by the state dental association
    d. elected to office by the state legislature

96. By state law the dentist employer of a dental hygienist is required to

    a. inspect all procedures
    b. inspect specified procedures
    c. be present during most procedures
    d. approve procedures in advance

97. The identification of a dental hygienist by name on business statements or stationery and the listing of her name on building directories or in telephone directories is

    a. seldom considered ethical
    b. occasionally considered ethical
    c. never considered unethical
    d. always considered unethical

98. The various state dental hygiene practice acts have specific areas of responsibility which are

    a. uniform in all states
    b. uniform in most states
    c. different in all states
    d. different in most states

99. The dental hygienist's scope of practice is directly regulated by the practice act of the state in which she

    a. is employed
    b. resides
    c. is licensed
    d. was educated

100. Amendments to dental hygiene practice acts are adopted by

    a. the state board of dental examiners
    b. the state legislature
    c. the governor's office
    d. the National Board of Dental Examiners

101. The dental hygienist would be performing an act of malpractice if

    a. the technical procedure was not indicated in the specific dental hygiene practice act

    b. treatment were rendered contrary to accepted procedure and injury resulted

    c. ordinary precautions were not exercised in giving treatment

    d. any of the above

102. Licensure laws have been designed basically for the express purpose of

    a. protecting the public health, safety, and welfare

    b. keeping incompetents from practicing

    c. giving status to the profession

    d. all of the above

103. The first state requiring dentists to pass a licensure examination was

    a. Georgia

    b. Connecticut

    c. Alabama

    d. Maryland

104. Legislative enactments regulating the practice of dentistry and dental hygiene are designed primarily to

    a. impose penalties for the violation of a law

    b. establish and maintain practice standards

    c. determine educational qualifications before practice

    d. improve the stature of the profession

105. Dental hygiene education is controlled by

    a. uniform state laws

    b. uniform state board regulations

    c. uniform education rulings

    d. none of the above

106. From a legal point of view, dental radiographs belong to

    a. only the dentist

    b. only the patient

    c. both the dentist and patient

    d. neither the dentist nor the patient

107. In the usual situation, an obligation to pay is created when a dental service is rendered because

    a. time and materials have been furnished

    b. a moral obligation exists

    c. a contract exists

    d. an ethical responsibility is involved

108. A malpractice statute of limitations restricts

    a. who may bring the action
    b. the conditions for which the action may be brought
    c. the time within which the action may be brought
    d. who may be the defendant in the action

109. A dentist is required to withhold the following taxes from employees' wages

    a. federal unemployment tax and federal income tax
    b. federal income tax and social security tax
    c. federal unemployment tax and self-employment tax
    d. federal income tax and workmen's compensation tax

110. Dental hygienists become members of the American Dental Hygienists' Association through

    a. district associations
    b. constituent associations
    c. regional associations
    d. any of the above associations

111. The organization responsible for determining whether a dental hygienist is guilty of malfeasance resides in the

    a constituent dental hygienists' association
    b. constituent dental associations
    c. state board of dental examiners
    d. National Board of Dental Examiners

112. Although there are many similarities between a profession and a business, the essential difference lies in the

    a. financial gains received
    b. quality of service rendered
    c. quantity of service rendered
    d. personal satisfaction received

113. The dental hygienist is permitted by law to expose radiographs in

    a. all states
    b. less than the majority of states
    c. more than half the states
    d. less than half the states

114. The order of employment most frequently considered by the dentist utilizing auxiliary services would be the

    a. dental assistant, dental hygienist, receptionist, and laboratory technician

    b. receptionist, dental assistant, dental hygienist, and laboratory technician

    c. receptionist, dental hygienist, dental assistant, and laboratory technician

    d. dental assistant, receptionist, dental hygienist, and laboratory technician

115. The problem of broken appointments in the dental office can be corrected by

    a. charging a minimum fee for each appointment

    b. educating the patient to the importance of each appointment

    c. collecting a fee for any broken appointment

    d. charging an additional fee for a broken appointment

116. Although the dental hygienist provides direct professional services for the patient, the dentist is obligated to

    a. re-examine only new patients

    b. re-examine only after the patients' original appointment

    c. re-examine all patients after each appointment

    d. re-examine every patient at the last appointment

117. To use a collecting agency for the collection of delinquent dental fees would be

    a. legally permissible but professionally unethical

    b. legally questionable and professionally unethical

    c. legally permissible and professionally ethical

    d. legally questionable but professionally ethical

118. Should a dental hygienist violate the principles of ethics of the professional society, the most severe discipline imposed by the society would be

    a. revocation of license by the society

    b. conviction of the individual by the society

    c. expulsion from membership by the society

    d. public censure by the society

119. If a dental hygienist violates the dental hygiene practice act, proceedings for suspension or revocation of licensure is the responsibility of

    a. the state dental hygiene society
    b. the state board of dental examiners
    c. the state dental society
    d. the state trial court

120. The highest standards of practice for the dental hygienist are contained in

    a. the dental hygiene practice act
    b. the code of ethics
    c. the dental practice act
    d. the dental hygiene oath

121. The concept "standard of care" infers that services rendered a patient have been

    a. reasonably performed
    b. perfectly performed
    c. precisely performed
    d. realistically performed

122. An act of malpractice has been committed when

    a. imperfect service is provided the patient
    b. a technical accident occurs and the patient is informed
    c. perfect service is guaranteed the patient
    d. a technical accident occurs and the patient is not informed

123. Legally the dentist is liable for the performance of auxiliary personnel under the doctrine of respondent superior, which implies

    a. responsibility for specific professional performances
    b. responsibility for limited professional performances
    c. responsibility for supervised professional performances
    d. responsibility for all professional performances

124. Although the dentist is liable under the respondent superior doctrine for auxiliary personnel, this ruling does not exonerate auxiliaries from being responsible for liability action through

    a. personal negligence
    b. professional negligence
    c. unintentional negligence
    d. unwarrantable negligence

125. To avoid being accused of technical assault, the dentist should obtain from the patient an agreement of

    a. written consent
    b. implied consent
    c. oral consent
    d. informed consent

126. The utilization of auxiliary personnel has been shown to be most extensive with the dental graduates during the years of the

    a. 1960
    b. 1950
    c. 1940
    d. 1930

127. Since it is advisable that an employment contract exist, this agreement should always be

    a. written to be legally binding
    b. mutually understood to be legally binding
    c. enforceable to be legally binding
    d. flexible to be legally binding

128. Every state dental practice act indicates in detail the acts which constitute the practice of dentistry and provides some exceptions for what is permitted by the dental hygienist. However, if an act comes within the definition of the practice of dentistry, but is not stated among the acts which are exceptions for the hygienist, this would be considered

    a. permissible if performed under the direction of the dentist
    b. unlawful even if performed under the direction of the dentist
    c. lawful if performed under the direction of the dentist
    d. acceptable if performed under the direction of the dentist

129. The concept "direction and control" means that the dentist

    a. must be in constant attendance when the dental hygienist is working
    b. can permit the dental hygienist to perform treatment at his discretion
    c. should be constantly available while the dental hygienist is working
    d. can permit the dental hygienist to provide services not specifically defined in the dental practice act

130. Requirements of dental hygiene licensure are included in the dental practice act, which specifies procedures that can be performed

    a. only by the dental hygienist
    b. by both the dental hygienist and dental assistant
    c. also by the dental assistant
    d. never by the dental hygienist

131. The dental hygienist is legally permitted to perform procedures

    a. sanctioned by an accredited program.
    b. stipulated by a board of dental examiners.
    c. stipulated by any board of dental examiners.
    d. sanctioned by a state statute.

132. Respondent superior implies "let the master answer," which would indicate that

    a. just the dentist is liable for an act of negligence
    b. just the dentist is liable for negligence committed by auxiliary personnel
    c. the dentist usually is liable for any act of negligence performed in the office
    d. the dentist always is liable for any act of negligence personally performed in the office

133. The general rule of law that is frequently referred to as the "Parol Evidence Rule" stipulates that

    a. the terms of the written agreement are binding and constitute a contract
    b. the terms of an oral agreement are binding and constitute a contract
    c. the terms of the written agreement are binding but the oral statements are variable
    d. the terms of either a or b are enforceable

134. When supplies are purchased on an open account, it means that payment is expected

    a. on delivery of the goods
    b. within 30 days of delivery of the goods
    c. upon rendering a statement of the account
    d. upon invoice rendered for the supplies

135. Malpractice insurance provides protection against

    a. liability for negligence
    b. liability for injury
    c. any and all claims
    d. the filing of lawsuits

136. Which of the following may be subject to malpractice actions?

    a. dentist
    b. dentist and dental hygienist
    c. dentist, dental hygienist, and dental assistant
    d. dentist, dental hygienist, dental assistant, and dental consultant

137. Premises liability insurance coverage extends to

    a. any individual who sustains an injury while on the premises by permission
    b. any patient who sustains a non-dental injury while on the premises
    c. any patient who sustains an injury while on the premises
    d. both b and c

138. In all probability, there is no technical assault

    a. when the patient's health is improved by the procedure
    b. when the dentist secures the implied consent of the patient to the procedure
    c. when the dentist secures the written consent of a blood relative of the patient
    d. if the need for additional procedures is established after a general anesthetic is administered

139. Should the dentist be threatened with a malpractice suit, it is advisable immediately to

    a. notify the insurance company and discuss the situation with the patient
    b. notify the insurance company and discuss the situation with the patient's attorney
    c. notify the insurance company and refrain from discussing the situation
    d. notify the insurance company and attempt to negotiate a settlement

140. The American Dental Hygienists' Association currently has group insurance policies covering the areas of

    a. accident, hospital, life, and income protection
    b. hospital, liability, life, and income protection
    c. liability, life, accident, and income protection
    d. accident, hospital, liability, and income protection

141. Financial arrangements for patient fees should always be

    a. discussed by the dentist
    b. discussed with the case presentation
    c. presented by a competent office employee
    d. presented by the business manager

142. A recall system is essential for any dental office and it has been determined from evaluation of different systems that the most effective approach is

    a. by direct telephoning at the time the appointment is needed
    b. by scheduling an appointment at the conclusion of treatment and later sending an appointment reminder
    c. by forwarding a reminder card with a scheduled appointment just prior to the recall appointment
    d. by forwarding a reminder card requesting the patient to telephone for a definite appointment to be scheduled

143. To better comprehend dental law the three basic services of American jurisprudence should be understood. These three general sources of American law are

    a. federal statutes, United States Constitution, state statutes
    b. federal statutes, state constitutions, state statutes
    c. federal statutes, state statutes, and judicial decisions
    d. federal statutes, judicial decisions, and the United States Constitution

144. When a licensed dental hygienist applies for a reciprocal license, the usual rule is that the licensing authority

    a. must issue the reciprocal license upon proof of prior licensure and payment of the required fee
    b. may issue the license at its discretion
    c. requires the cancellation of the prior license
    d. must accept or reject the application

145. State statutes are applicable just within the geographical confines of each respective state but are subject to

    a. judge-made law
    b. common law
    c. the United States Constitution
    d. both a and b

146. The validity of common or judge-made law extends

   a. just within the jurisdiction of the judge rendering the decision
   b. to all courts in the state where the judge rendered the decision
   c. only to federal court cases
   d. only to state court cases

147. Dentistry is controlled through the individual state legislation which is provided by a statute known as

   a. judicial power
   b. legislative power
   c. police power
   d. executive power

148. The statute that governs dentist-patient relationship would be contained in

   a. the dental practice act
   b. common law documents
   c. federal legislation
   d. all of the above

149. Boards of dental examiners are created by the

   a. United States Congress
   b. state legislatures
   c. state dental societies
   d. American Dental Association

150. One facet of professionalism is continuing education, which is specified in the American Dental Hygienists' Association

   a. Constitution
   b. Bylaws
   c. Principles of Ethics
   d. Licensure

151. The governing agency of a profession is inherently influenced primarily through the

   a. council on dental education
   b. accrediting committee
   c. boards of dental examiners
   d. professional societies

152. Advertising by the dental hygienist is

   a. always considered unethical
   b. usually considered unethical
   c. seldom considered ethical
   d. occasionally considered ethical

153. The utilization of directories by a dental hygienist is

    a. never considered ethical
    b. seldom considered unethical
    c. restrictively considered ethical
    d. occasionally considered unethical

154. There has been considerable concern regarding the dental hygienist's professional use of recall notices, personal letterheads or announcement cards. It is generally felt that

    a. if used in any instance it would be ethically unacceptable
    b. if used with the consent of the superior it would be ethically acceptable
    c. if used in conjunction with the superior it would be ethically acceptable
    d. if used advisedly by the superior it would be ethically acceptable

155. The dental hygienist should be aware of the proper protocol in using office door lettering and signs. The principles of ethics of the American Dental Hygienists' Association indicates that this action is

    a. never considered ethical
    b. occasionally considered ethical
    c. seldom considered unethical
    d. frequently considered unethical

156. After the dental hygienist has become licensed the initials RDH are

    a. never permissible if used commercially
    b. always permissible if used commercially
    c. occasionally permissible if used patronizingly
    d. frequently permissible if used patronizingly

157. Should an ethical situation arise, the judicial procedure ought to be initially managed through

    a. component level channels
    b. national level channels
    c. constituent level channels
    d. district level channels

158. The dental hygienist who practices contrary to the requirements of a dental hygiene practice act could be committing

    a. a misdemeanor
    b. a felony
    c. a tort
    d. all of the above

159. Historically the dental hygiene professional development can be attributed to the dentist's concern in

    a. pedodontics and operative dentistry
    b. periodontics and preventive dentistry
    c. pedodontics and preventive dentistry
    d. periodontics and operative dentistry

160. The original dental hygiene program was established for the purpose of providing dental hygienists to

    a. philanthropic dental clinics
    b. public school systems
    c. pedodontic dental clinics
    d. private dental practitioners

161. Although the majority of dental hygienists are graduated from accredited schools, it is still acceptable to receive dental hygiene training by preceptorship in the states of

    a. Georgia and Louisiana
    b. Alabama and Louisiana
    c. Alabama and Georgia
    d. none of the above

162. A survey of dental hygienists revealed that the majority had

    a. 10 years of experience or less
    b. 15 years of experience or less
    c. 20 years of experience or less
    d. 25 years of experience or less

163. Factors that most frequently contribute to the choice of a career in dental hygiene, listed in the order of their significance, are

    a. experience as a dental assistant, encouragement of family dentist, and good salary and working conditions
    b. good salary and working conditions, encouragement of family dentist, and experience as dental assistant
    c. family dentist, experience as dental assistant, and good salary and working conditions
    d. encouragement of family dentist, good salary and working conditions, and experience as dental assistant

164. From a selected study concerning the various forms of compensation received by the dental hygienist, it was revealed that the majority were paid

    a. both a salary and commission
    b. a commission only
    c. a straight salary
    d. a salary with a bonus

165. The dental hygienist is employed primarily by the private practitioner who concentrates essentially on

    a. general dentistry
    b pedodontic dentistry
    c. periodontic dentistry
    d. prosthetic dentistry

166. A questionnaire has disclosed that the majority of dentists employing dental hygienists are between the age of

    a. 30 to 39 years
    b. 40 to 49 years
    c. 50 to 59 years
    d. 60 to 69 years

167. The American Dental Hygienists' Association is comprised of constituent representation from all but one state in the

    a. south central section of the country
    b. east central section of the country
    c. north central section of the country
    d. west central section of the country

168. The American Dental Hygienists' Association motto which is a part of the official seal is

    a. devotion
    b. service
    c. care
    d. courtesy

169. Historically, the dental hygienist became first organized professionally on the

    a. component level
    b. district level
    c. constituent level
    d. national level

170. There are several American Dental Hygienists' Association membership classifications, but the one awarded every outgoing president is known as

    a. honorary
    b. life
    c. retired
    d. active

171. In 1947, the Council on Dental Education of the American Dental Association and the House of Delegates of the American Dental Association accepted standards for dental hygiene programs known as

    a. required standards of education of the dental hygienist
    b. basic standards of education of the dental hygienist
    c. fundamental standards of education of the dental hygienist
    d. minimum standards of education of the dental hygienist

172. At the national meeting the trustee conducts a session with the delegates and alternates regarding issues to be considered before the House of Delegates, which is referred to as a

    a. caucas
    b. reference
    c. conference
    d. referendum

173. Every formally structured organization functions by a constitution which should be

    a. complex in form and contain only provisions that are expected to be permanent
    b. complex in form and contain only provisions that are expected to be temporary
    c. simple in form and contain only provisions that are expected to be temporary
    d. simple in form and contain only provisions that are expected to be permanent

174. During the national meeting the House of Delegates conducts a reviewing session of the different submitted reports and resolutions which is known as a

    a. special committee hearing
    b. reference committee hearing
    c. standing committee hearing
    d. referendum committee hearing

175. By-laws of an organization provide for

    a. operational rules and regulations
    b. parliamentary guide rulings
    c. responsibility of officers
    d. all of the above functions

176. The presiding officer of an organization has various observances to consider while conducting a meeting which would include

    a. referring to the chair as "I"
    b. entering into a discussion after relinquishing the chair
    c. remaining partisan in attitude
    d. both b and c

177. An organization desiring to transact a specific item of business brings the matter before the group through a main motion which is brought to a vote by requesting for the

    a. privilege
    b. decision
    c. question
    d. discussion

178. Any organization requesting an individual to serve in the absence of the regular officer would be officiating in the capacity of being

    a. pro tem
    b. ad-hoc
    c. ex-officio
    d. none of the above

179. The function of a parliamentarian during the meeting is to provide

    a. rulings
    b. advice
    c. decisions
    d. all of the above

180. Legally an organization can officially transact business only when there are enough members present to form a

    a. quota
    b. quotient
    c. quittance
    d. quorum

181. Minutes of a meeting should

    a. include discussion of every motion
    b. omit the statement "respectfully submitted" at the end of the minutes
    c. include mention of all motions
    d. include the name of the seconder of a motion

182. An organization can become incorporated under the laws of the state in which it exists, and this is advisable because incorporation provides

    a. a legality for ownership of property
    b. exclusive rights to its name
    c. protection for the membership in case of suit
    d. all of the above

183. When an individual is elected through common consent, he is said to be elected by

    a. acclamation
    b. unanimous vote
    c. acceptance
    d. unappealable decision

184. When used at the conclusion of a meeting, the expression "sine die" means

    a. temporary adjournment without a specific time for reconvening
    b. temporary adjournment with a specific time for reconvening
    c. adjournment without a specific time for reconvening
    d. adjournment with a specific time for reconvening

185. In structuring a resolution the section beginning whereas is known as the

    a. introduction
    b. preamble
    c. motion
    d. foundation

186. Final authority for official American Dental Hygienists' Association transactions are the responsibility of the

    a. Board of Trustees
    b. Executive Officers
    c. House of Delegates
    d. both a and b

187. A trustee is permitted to serve for

    a. two alternate three-year terms
    b. two consecutive three-year terms
    c. two consecutive six-year terms
    d. two alternate six-year terms

188. The trustee is the official liaison representative for

    a. district members on the Board of Trustees
    b. component members on the Board of Trustees
    c. constituent members on the Board of Trustees
    d. all of the above

189. Reference committee sessions are conducted

    a. to review previously submitted resolutions
    b. to vote upon previously submitted resolutions
    c. to eliminate discussion at the House of Delegates
    d. to clarify discussion at the general meetings

190. American Dental Hygienists Association reference committee sessions are

    a. open meetings for all delegates
    b. closed meetings for select delegates
    c. open meetings for all members
    d. closed meetings for select members

191. The House of Delegates establishes policies by either the acceptance or rejection of

    a. recommendations
    b. reports
    c. referendums
    d. resolutions

192. Every constituent is privileged to have representation at the House of Delegates through selection of an individual or individuals known as a

    a. representative
    b. proxy
    c. delegate
    d. trustee

193. The terms licensed and certified are frequently used interchangeably, but there is

    a. a significant legal differentiation
    b. an insignificant legal differentiation
    c. no legal differentiation
    d. a varied legal differentiation

194. The major portion of all activities comprising the American Dental Hygienists' Association is assumed by the

    a. officers
    b. trustees
    c. committees
    d. chairman

195. Scheduling of appointments is an important factor in establishing a well managed office and therefore it is preferable to

    a. provide a rigid maximum time since this arrangement is economically advantageous
    b. provide a flexible minimum time since this arrangement is economically advantageous
    c. provide a flexible maximum time since this arrangement is economically advantageous
    d. provide a rigid minimum time since this arrangement is economically advantageous

196. Change in any dental hygiene licensure enactments is within the power of the state

    a. legislature
    b. dental examiners
    c. dental society
    d. governor

197. The number of dental hygienists graduated each year is approximately

    a. 1500
    b. 2000
    c. 2500
    d. 3000

198. Boards of dental examiners have the responsibility of

    a. protecting the public from incompetents
    b. determining the continuing competency of practitioners
    c. providing continuing education programs
    d. all of the above

199. Licensure for the dental hygienist requires examination in both theory and practice by

    a. more than half the states
    b. less than half the states
    c. few states
    d. all states

200. The American Dental Hygienists' Association structure and specific regulations by which its affairs are governed appear in the

    a. constitution
    b. bylaws
    c. charter
    d. articles of incorporation

ANSWERS

1. c	37. d	73. c	109. b
2. b	38. b	74. c	110. b
3. c	39. c	75. d	111. c
4. c	40. d	76. c	112. b
5. b	41. c	77. c	113. c
6. d	42. c	78. d	114. d
7. b	43. d	79. d	115. b
8. a	44. a	80. c	116. c
9. d	45. c	81. a	117. c
10. b	46. b	82. a	118. c
11. c	47. c	83. d	119. b
12. a	48. b	84. b	120. b
13. c	49. d	85. b	121. a
14. c	50. b	86. c	122. d
15. c	51. b	87. b	123. d
16. a	52. b	88. d	124. a
17. b	53. a	89. c	125. d
18. b	54. b	90. b	126. b
19. b	55. c	91. c	127. b
20. b	56. a	92. d	128. b
21. b	57. c	93. b	129. c
22. b	58. c	94. b	130. a
23. d	59. d	95. a	131. d
24. b	60. a	96. a	132. c
25. d	61. d	97. d	133. a
26. b	62. c	98. b	134. c
27. c	63. b	99. a	135. a
28. b	64. d	100. b	136. d
29. d	65. c	101. d	137. a
30. b	66. c	102. d	138. b
31. c	67. b	103. c	139. c
32. d	68. b	104. b	140. d
33. c	69. b	105. d	141. c
34. b	70. a	106. a	142. b
35. b	71. b	107. c	143. c
36. c	72. d	108. c	144. b

145. c	159. c	173. d	187. b
146. a	160. b	174. b	188. d
147. c	161. c	175. d	189. a
148. b	162. a	176. b	190. c
149. b	163. a	177. c	191. d
150. c	164. c	178. a	192. c
151. d	165. a	179. b	193. a
152. a	166. a	180. d	194. c
153. c	167. c	181. b	195. c
154. c	168. b	182. d	196. a
155. b	169. c	183. a	197. a
156. a	170. b	184. c	198. a
157. c	171. d	185. b	199. d
158. d	172. a	186. c	200. b

REFERENCES

1. American Dental Hygienists' Association: *Constitution, By Laws and Principles of Ethics.* Chicago, 1962.
2. American Dental Hygienists' Association: *Structure and Function of the American Dental Hygienists' Association.* Chicago, 1965.
3. Campbell, R.: *The Dental Hygienist in Private Practice.* Dubuque, W. C. Brown Co., 1964.
4. Carnahan, C. W.: *Carnahan's The Dentist and the Law.* 2nd Ed. William W. Howard and Alex L. Parks, St. Louis, C. V. Mosby Co., 1965.
5. Hollinshead, B. S.: *Survey of Dentistry: The Final Report.* Washington, D.C., American Council on Education, pp. 182–238, 1961.
6. Sarner, H.: *The Business Management of Dental Practice.* Philadelphia, W. B. Saunders Co., 1966.
7. Sarner, H.: *Dental Jurisprudence.* Philadelphia, W. B. Saunders Co., 1963.
8. Steele, P. F.: *Dimensions of Dental Hygiene.* Philadelphia, Lea & Febiger, XII, 1966.
9. Stinaff, R. K.: *Dental Practice Administration.* 2nd Ed., St. Louis, C. V. Mosby Co., 1964.
10. Suthers, M. H.: *Primer in Parliamentary Procedure.* 5th Ed., Chicago, Dartnell, 1963.